PRAISE FOR
COMPLETE WITHOUT KIDS

"Having reviewed Dr. Walker's book, I'm very excited for the childfree community. Her expertise, research, and personal experience shine through. Her book will be a necessary read for anyone exploring the childfree/childless topic, whether out of curiosity or personal choices regarding such an important decision. I hope more young people will explore the idea of becoming childfree, in addition to examining their own reasons for wanting to become a parent. *Complete Without Kids* provides a timely look into the reasons individuals become either child*free* or child*less*. Insightful, well-researched, and compassionate."

—Cara Swann, author and freelance writer

"Like becoming a parent, 'childfree' living is an option best left to each individual to decide. Dr. Walker's guide is a wonderful tool, whether you are 'childfree' by choice, circumstance, or happenstance, to help you understand you are not alone. You will see yourself in this book."

—Linda McCarthy, executive director, Mt. Baker Planned Parenthood

"Helpful, supportive, and thought-provoking are terms I would use to describe *Complete Without Kids*. I recommend it to those who are considering or who have embarked upon a childfree life for whatever reasons. Dr. Walker's own story and those of the people she interviewed lets childfree people know that they are in good company."

—Dr. Karen M. Aronoff, PsyD, clinical psychologist

"As a young adult entering a phase in my life when questions and pressures regarding future choices are plentiful, I found that Dr. Walker's book provides a much needed exploration of childfree living. By incorporating real-life accounts with psychological insight, Dr. Walker sheds an important awareness on a population of families that are often overlooked because they do not have children. While transitioning into adulthood during a time of constant global economic and environmental concern, it is critical that upcoming generations are empowered with a sense of responsibility and choice, which is one of the many ways that Dr. Walker's book is a success."

—Anna Wolff, psychology student, Western Washington University

"I do not want kids! I do want . . . mega money, vast vacations, . . . freedom, and of course, a copy of this book. It takes a very special person not to make babies . . . unlike [most people who] only thereafter realize the lifelong ramifications and responsibilities."

—Christopher M. Puzzele, Esq., creator of IDoNOTWantKids.com

COMPLETE
WITHOUT
KIDS

ELLEN L. WALKER, PH.D.

COMPLETE
WITHOUT
KIDS

AN INSIDER'S GUIDE TO CHILDFREE LIVING
BY CHOICE OR BY CHANCE

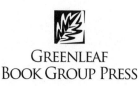

GREENLEAF
BOOK GROUP PRESS

This book is intended as a reference volume only, not as a therapeutic manual. The information given here is designed to help you make informed decisions. It is not intended as a substitute for any treatment that may have been recommended by a mental health care professional.

Published by Greenleaf Book Group Press
Austin, Texas
www.gbgpress.com

Distributed by Greenleaf Book Group LLC

For ordering information or special discounts for bulk purchases, please contact Greenleaf Book Group LLC at PO Box 91869, Austin, TX 78709, 512.891.6100.

Design and composition by Greenleaf Book Group LLC and Alex Head
Cover design by Greenleaf Book Group LLC and Dan Pitts

Publisher's Cataloging-In-Publication Data
(Prepared by The Donohue Group, Inc.)
Walker, Ellen L. (Ellen Lind), 1960-
    Complete without kids : an insider's guide to childfree living by choice or by chance / Ellen L. Walker. — 2nd ed.
        p. ; cm.
    First edition published as: I don't have kids : the guide to childfree living / Ellen Walker, c2010.
    Includes bibliographical references.
    ISBN: 978-1-60832-073-8
    1. Childlessness—Psychological aspects. 2. Childlessness—Social aspects. I. Title.
II. I don't have kids
HQ755.8 .W35 2011
306.87   2010932566

Part of the Tree Neutral® program, which offsets the number of trees consumed in the production and printing of this book by taking proactive steps, such as planting trees in direct proportion to the number of trees used: www.treeneutral.com

TreeNeutral®

Printed in the United States of America on acid-free paper

10 11 12 13 14 15   10 9 8 7 6 5 4 3 2 1

Second Edition

CONTENTS

PREFACE

Complete Without Kids: An Insider's Guide to Childfree Living by Choice or by Chance is a project that began over two years ago in the pages of my personal journal. As I talked with others about the idea, I received much encouragement, simply because of the uniqueness of the topic and the slim choice of books available for adults who are childfree or those contemplating whether to have kids. It was not until November 2008, however, that I took a day-long writing course and shared with a small group of fellow dreamers that I wanted to write this book.

What followed was a chance meeting with a woman who introduced me to her editor and writing coach, Brooke Warner. Brooke walked me through every step, helping me learn a whole new style of writing, quite the opposite of the psychological reports that I craft every day in my clinical practice. The process has, of course, been energizing but also frustrating. I am very thankful to Brooke for her patience and ongoing support over the past year.

I am also grateful to the women, men, and couples who came forward to participate in my interviews. I appreciate your honesty and willingness to share your most personal stories with me. Conducting those interviews and reading the written responses from participants was truly the most delightful part of this entire process.

I would not have been able to complete the book without the ongoing support of my husband, Chris Portman. Chris listened to hours of brainstorming and encouraged me to write rather than play on weekend mornings. He has also supported me in taking time away from my day job to complete the project.

I am appreciative, as always, of my parents, Marjorie and George Walker, who believe in me and have stuck by me from day one.

INTRODUCTION

I thought the whole baby thing was behind me, but just when I least expected it, babylust hit me. It was the summer of 2006, and I'd just moved into a small apartment with my new husband Chris. Chris is a psychologist, like me, a decade older than me, and the first *father* I'd ever had a relationship with. When we got together, I was forty-five years old and feeling at peace with the idea that I would not have children. I had created a rich and busy life for myself with my clinical psychology practice, my dog Bella, and lots of friends and activities. Because Chris's children were grown and on their own, I never gave a second thought to the possibility that observing him interact with them would cause me grief. So it came as a big surprise the first time I heard Chris on the telephone say, "I love you, son," and I felt a sudden sharp pain in my heart. The ache only intensified when we talked more about his children and he shared that being a dad was one of the most fulfilling parts of his life. I began to feel a huge sadness in the realization that no one would ever call me "Mom" and that I'd never say, "I love you, son" to a child of my own. For the first time, I began to question my decision not to have children, and I wondered if I'd made a huge mistake. I knew that at age forty-five, it was not too late, but I'd need to act quickly if I wanted to try to get pregnant.

Over that first summer together, I witnessed more of these loving interactions between Chris and his children, and my emotions churned. It seemed that everywhere I went there were pregnant women and adorable children. Chris and I had quite a few tearful discussions, but he was clear that he didn't want to have another child. Gradually, after weeks of tears, writing, talking, and contemplating, my emotions began to settle, and I was able to see more objectively what becoming a mother would mean for me, both positively and negatively. I was able to understand why I had gravitated toward a childfree life and why shifting gears at this point would be a mistake for me. I also knew that I wanted to have Chris as my lifelong playmate, not as a co-parent in raising a child. I began to once again embrace my identity as *childfree* and, for the first time in my life, I started to actively seek out other childfree adults. I had a curiosity about these peers—I wanted to hear about their experiences, to know if they had also struggled in arriving at their decision. I began to discover that, while many childfree adults have strong feelings about the topic, most have not talked much about it and are eager to do so. On a couple of occasions, I found myself in the corner of a crowded party whispering with another childfree adult as if we were secret members of a special club. We felt excitement and validation in our connection.

As I began to contemplate my personal experience and to ask others about theirs, *Complete Without Kids: An Insider's Guide to Childfree Living by Choice or by Chance* started to take shape. I sought out literature on the subject and was surprised to find only a handful of books published over the past twenty years, most of which have a seemingly anti-children agenda and strongly promote a childfree life. One of my primary goals was to examine childfree living from a neutral position, in a way that would allow readers to see that this life choice is like any other, with both positive and negative aspects. I wanted to hear from those who might have had kids had their lives taken a different course (whom I have defined as Childfree by Happenstance), those who are happily childfree (Childfree by Choice), and also those who are sad about not having had kids (Childfree by Circumstance).

Another goal of this book was to present an accurate picture of the childfree adult experience for younger generations, as some youths are questioning their desire to become parents but continue to feel pressure to do so because society strongly celebrates babies and traditional families.

As a psychologist, my favorite role is listening to my clients tell their life stories. Something magical happens during this process, as they are able to see more clearly how they have arrived at their current place in life and where they want to go from there. *Complete Without Kids* tells these stories shared by childfree adults and examines the behind-the-scenes factors that influenced their journeys. Because I enjoy journaling and have had my own personal journey in exploring being childfree, I chose to include my experiences along with those of the people I interviewed.

In addition to exploring the paths taken to arrive at a life without kids, I also wanted to satisfy my own curiosity about other childfree adults. I wanted to discover whether or not we are truly different as a group—in our personalities and our daily lives—from those who are parents. I recognized that childfree adults face a unique set of problems simply due to living in a family-focused society (somewhat like being left-handed in a right-handed world), and I hoped to identify some of these issues and to provide suggestions about how to cope with them in a healthy way.

While contemplating writing a book on living childfree, I deliberated terminology, starting out using the word *childless* but feeling a negative charge whenever I said it aloud. *Childlessness* felt like a grieving or a missing out on something essential. So instead, I chose to use the term *childfree*, which for me implies a life in which we're free to put our energies into endeavors other than raising children. *Childfree* as opposed to *childless* also demonstrates the positive feeling I have about my own personal choice, without in any way criticizing the choice of those who have decided to have children.

When I began to put out the word that I was conducting interviews for my book, I started by approaching friends and relatives who are childfree. Some of these individuals never responded to my invitation to talk about their experiences, and I realized that for many, being childfree is a true source of pain that may be best left untouched. On the other hand, I found that many of my personal feelings and experiences were shared by others, many of whom had never voiced their own feelings aloud and were eager to do so. Those who responded are a diverse group of men, women, and couples; straight and gay; from across the United States; ranging in age from their mid-thirties to ninety. To protect their privacy, I have changed names and other identifying information. As you read their stories you will see that, as is often the case with major life choices, one feels a loss for the path not taken, and an uncertainty about whether the best decision was made. I feel privileged to have been allowed to hear these life journeys, rich and filled with twists and turns.

I invite you to join others and me in exploring the journey and embracing the destination of a childfree life!

CHAPTER 1
THE PATH TO CHILDFREE

"I think we have to make choices in life, and the choice for me
was to embrace all person-kind rather than concentrate on one
single individual . . . The universal is what I've selected."
—Leo Buscaglia

How often do you have the experience of meeting someone new and being asked, "Do you have children?" Most women my age would respond to this common question with a simple "Yes," which would be followed by a dialogue about her children's names, ages, and activities. It's interesting to note, however, what happens when I say, "No, I don't have kids." My response is most often followed by silence because people don't know what to say. Should they ask about my reasons for not having had kids? If I were ten years younger, they might want to know if children were in my plans. The conversation instantly feels overly personal, and I usually break the silence by making a reassuring comment about being fine with not having had kids, and then asking them about their own children. With the shift to this safer topic, the feeling of relief is almost palpable. I can only imagine how this kind of conversation must feel for a woman who has tried to have children but has been unsuccessful, or someone who had a child but lost him or her through some tragic life circumstances. Even a childfree adult who is content with her decision may wonder if the other person thinks she dislikes children—or, she may be reminded of her own ambivalence about not having kids. The reality is that childfree adults are like any other minority group, in that while there are myriad reasons behind our childfree status, we share the common experience of often feeling misunderstood and left out.

As you will read in the pages ahead, there is no one type of childfree adult, and our behind-the-scenes stories are often complex and always personal. Perhaps the largest group includes adults who might have had kids had their lives taken a different route. For them, it just never happened. A second category is made up of those who report that they always knew they didn't want to have kids, and yet another group is comprised of those who wanted to but couldn't have children and are grieving this absence in their lives. Although separated into three groups—Childfree by Happenstance, Childfree by Choice, and Childfree by Circumstance—the lines between categories are often blurred. As with any life situation, there are positives and negatives, joys and pains associated with being childfree.

Childfree by Happenstance: It Just Never Happened

"For me, the price was that I never married and never had children because there was never time. And if I had ever decided to do any of that it would have taken Fleetwood Mac off for two years and the band would have broken up. So that wasn't even acceptable. That wasn't even a choice."
—Stevie Nicks, Fleetwood Mac

Many childfree adults, including myself, ended up not being a parent due to situational factors and didn't really spend much time contemplating the decision. I grew up in a traditional Southern home where my family expected that I'd go off to college, earn my "Mrs." degree, and start a family right away. My older brother married his high school sweetheart and then dutifully began the process of starting a family. Following in his footsteps never seemed like an option for me—I wanted to choose my own path in life. Like all the other girls I grew up with, I babysat, but I would only agree to watch children whose parents put them to bed before I arrived. I was seldom around babies. By the time I had my first real boyfriend, I was in college and into being a free spirit. I didn't want to be held back by anything. Now here I am, forty-eight years old, and I've never even changed a diaper!

As I entered my mid-thirties, I occasionally wondered if I would regret not having children. I felt pressure, mostly from myself, to produce a grandchild for my parents. It was also around this time that two of my best friends unexpectedly became pregnant. But the years went by and my life was busy, fun, and fulfilling!

> "I grew up in a traditional Southern home where my family expected that I'd go off to college, earn my "Mrs." degree, and start a family right away."

I kept forgetting to take the time to actually decide whether or not I wanted to have children, and the men in my life clearly stated that they did not want to have kids. These factors combined with not having a strong maternal urge, and as the years passed, I became childfree almost by default. I recall dating a couple of men when I was in my mid-thirties who talked about wanting to be dads, and I'm certain that, had one of these relationships progressed to something more permanent, I would have become a mother and I'd likely have enjoyed that role tremendously.

Many childfree adults, including some who shared their stories with me, report having this same sense: that they might have had children had their lives taken a different direction, such as marrying someone who really wanted kids, or becoming pregnant unexpectedly. Diane, a forty-three-year-old accountant, lives with her partner Patrick in a large home in the country with their two dogs.

Diane and I met in their sunny living room overlooking the neatly landscaped property, and she told me about her life. "We didn't actually make a conscious decision to be childfree. Early in our relationship we talked about having kids *later*, though we never defined what that meant. The topic came up from time to time, but it simply wasn't a priority. Our most serious discussion came about six years ago, after we'd been together for thirteen years, when our close friends decided to have a child." Diane laughed, and added, "At that point we came to the conclusion that we just weren't thrilled about the idea of having a teenager at fifty-five. At times during our relationship I've felt I made a mistake by not having kids, but through the years, I've grown very comfortable with our life, as has Patrick. I don't feel like our lives are incomplete because we really do the things we love to do. I haven't taken any steps to make peace with the decision—it simply became the right decision over time."

"Pondering being childfree took me back—mine was sort of a non-decision decision."

Diane and Patrick were so busy living their lives that they didn't notice that there might have been a missing piece until their friends talked about having a child. They then considered their options and agreed that they were happy with their life as it was. If anything, the review of where they were and where they wanted to go may have led to a heightened awareness of the kind of life they wanted to create for themselves, a full and rich adult world centered around work and play.

Diane and Patrick's story is not unique—many of my interviewees' lives have been filled with twists and turns, starting out intending to have kids but then experiencing life events that prevented it. I met with Trish, a sixty-five-year-old divorced psychotherapist, in her office on a Friday afternoon. "Pondering being childfree took me back—mine was sort of a non-decision decision," she told me. "I grew up in a family where children were appreciated, and there were lots of cousins around all the time. I married in 1964 and was among the first to use the Pill. After Gary finished college and got a job, we decided that it was a good time to start a family, and so I got off the Pill. Nothing happened for years, and then, by surprise, I found out that I was pregnant. We were delighted, but then I miscarried about seven months along. Unfortunately, Gary and I didn't know how to talk to each other about the miscarriage, and this likely resulted in the breakdown of our relationship. We divorced two years later. By that point, I was working at a mental health clinic and my coworkers encouraged me to go back to college for a master's degree. I did so, and then began working as a psychotherapist. During those years, in my mid-thirties, my life was all about finding out what I wanted to do. I had lots of people around me giving me support and validation for being smart. When I was thirty-five years old, I ended up having ovarian cancer and had a total hysterectomy. I was on my own, and so having a child wasn't on my mind anyway. Two of my close friends were mothers, and one of these women told me that she didn't feel like she was a good mother. I was able to mother her in a sense and to support her in her role as a parent. I've also been very active with my sister's children since the time they were born. I've had the good part of having kids around without the diapers."

Trish's story left an impression on me. I wondered how a person who has experienced such great pain and loss in her life—with her miscarriage, divorce, cancer, and hysterectomy—has not only healed from her pain in a fairly brief time, but also has become involved with nieces and nephews while mentoring and supporting friends who are struggling in their roles as parents. I hear about other women who have had miscarriages and then do not want to be around kids at all due to the pain it causes. They appear to be stuck in the trauma of their experience, unable to move ahead in their life. Why has Trish been able to embrace her life as it has unfolded? One likely explanation is that she was able to grieve her losses fully and to accept where she was in her life. She then was able to evaluate what her mothering needs were and to identify healthy ways to meet these through her experience of counseling others, supporting friends who were moms, and being involved in the lives of her nieces and nephews. Trish has all the signs of a psychologically healthy adult who is able to respond to life by making choices about things that are in her control, accepting what she cannot control or change, and identifying her needs and finding healthy ways to meet them.

On a sunny Saturday afternoon, I met with Jackie in my home. She told me that she would have liked to be a mom had things been different for her. Jackie is a fifty-year-old paralegal who has never been married and hasn't had a serious romantic relationship for years. She shared, "I always thought I'd grow up and have children, but it just didn't happen. Now I realize the level of responsibility that having a child involves. A child must be put first—even before your marriage. I pretty much raised my younger brother and sister, and so I had some of the experiences of child rearing when I was young. Because of this, I knew that I didn't like it—yet I still assumed that I'd marry and have kids."

Jackie expressed frustration with parents who complain about their children, saying that she recently got together with her sister, who has a seventeen-year-old daughter. "I sat there and listened to my sister go on and on about how irresponsible her daughter is, having friends over and not cleaning up after themselves. I know that if I were to challenge my sister on why she chose to have a child, she would point out the good things, like how wonderful it was to tuck her daughter in at night and to comfort her when she skinned her knee. If I heard those memories, I know I'd feel sad. I sometimes think about how nice it would be to hear a child say, 'I love you, Mommy,' but there's a huge amount of heartbreak to deal with, too. It means a lot to know that when I come home at night I can spend my time the way I want to rather than being obligated to come home and turn my attention to another person. I've always been agitated by noise and crowds and I don't think I'd get over it, even if I had children."

Jackie's story is typical of a childfree adult who has mixed emotions about her childfree status. She intended to be a mom, but it didn't happen for her. She also understands that there are positives about not being a parent, and she seems to have reached a place of relative peace with her situation. As Jackie talked about her need for quiet and calm, I thought about how much enjoyment I get from spending time in my home without noise or clutter. I wondered if most childfree adults prefer calm and quiet, or if Jackie and I were experiencing *cognitive dissonance,* a psychological term coined by Leon Festinger described as the uncomfortable feeling that results when a person holds two contradictory attitudes or beliefs at the same time.[1] This discomfort can cause us to change, justify, or rationalize our attitudes, beliefs, and behaviors. In the example of someone like Jackie or myself, it makes sense that we would claim to prefer a calm, quiet environment, because that's the environment we've cultivated in our homes for our entire adult lives without children. Had we become parents, however, we might claim that we prefer the lively chaos of a full house.

> *Cognitive dissonance* is a psychological term described as the uncomfortable feeling that results when a person holds two contradictory attitudes or beliefs at the same time.

Denise, also single, is a sixty-one-year-old psychiatric office manager, who drove up from Seattle to meet with me in my home. Like most women, she assumed as a child that she would have her own family someday. She grew up with three siblings, a father who worked, and a mother who was a homemaker. She noted, "I always thought I'd stay home, like Mom did, and raise children. I went to university to become a teacher—so I'd have something to fall back on. I got married at age twenty, and because my husband was still in school, I needed to work to support us. I became a secretary, and I thought that I'd just be working until my husband finished college and that we'd start a family at that point. He was in school for four years, and during that time we began to have marital problems. I also learned about the mental health history in his family. When I got a job at our local mental health clinic, I found out more about mental illness, including my husband's depression."

Denise told me how, along the way, she kept waiting for that irresistible urge to have a baby that people talk about, but it never happened for her. She was waiting to sense the biological clock that is discussed more in depth in chapter 2. "I wonder if my knowledge of genetics and mental illness played a part in suppressing that urge," she pondered. "I decided that I didn't want a child coming from that gene pool, nor did I want to end up being a single mom or the primary breadwinner and caretaker for our child. My husband and I divorced when I was thirty-eight, and I didn't trust myself to choose someone who was mentally healthy. I assumed that my lack of longing for a child was a sign that perhaps I should simply not have kids." I asked Denise if, looking back on her life, she felt that she made the right decision for herself. She shared that not having kids has meant that she has had time and energy to nurture others, including the doctors she works for and her large circle of friends. Like Trish and Jackie, Denise seemed to be a person with the ability to accept and embrace life in a healthy way as opposed to living it with regrets. As Denise talked, I recognized one of Sigmund Freud's coping tools at work for her: rationalization.[2] This involves explaining losses and coming up with logical reasons for them; we even convince ourselves that we did not want to have these things anyway. By this point in her life, Denise may not even be able to

> Rationalization involves explaining losses and coming up with logical reasons for them; we even convince ourselves that we did not want to have these things anyway.

separate out whether she would have truly preferred to be a mother as opposed to being childfree. I suspect that, had she met a wonderful man who was emotionally healthy and wanted to have children with her, Denise would have experienced a maternal drive. Since this situation did not occur, nothing sparked the yearning. There's nothing she can do to change the way her life has unfolded, and so she has decided that this is the way it was naturally supposed to be for her.

Carrie, a fifty-one-year-old married medical biller, met with me at my office on a brisk Saturday morning. As she began to talk, she shared, "Steven and I spent last night on our sailboat, as we often do during the spring and summer. It's fun and relaxing to sleep on the boat, even if we don't take it out. We have several friends who also have boats, so it's a real social scene." Carrie was born and raised in a small Idaho town where her parents still live, and she grew up in a traditional family with a stay-at-home mother and a father who worked. She mused, "I thought growing up that I would have children. I got married when I was twenty-one, and I assumed that we'd start a family, but when I brought it up with my husband, he said, '*You've* got to grow up first and then you can have one!' We were married for seven years, and he had several affairs, which led to our divorce. I was single for a couple of years before Steven and I got together. Steven had three children who lived with his first wife in another state, and when I told my mother about his kids, she said, 'Run for the hills!'" Carrie laughed as she continued, "After Steven and I got married, I thought for a brief time, perhaps a month, that we should have kids. Then I said to myself, 'Oh, forget about it.' I didn't really ever make a firm decision about whether or not to have kids,

> "I got married when I was twenty-one and I assumed that we'd start a family, but when I brought it up with my husband, he said, 'You've got to grow up first and then you can have one!'"

but because I never felt a strong desire to do so, it simply never happened. Steven would have been willing to have a child with me had I really wanted this. I continued to take the Pill until a couple of years ago when Steven had a vasectomy." Carrie sighed, "I always envied people who were sure about their decision, because I've always been ambivalent. I don't think I ever really wanted to have them, but I wonder what I've missed out on."

It's probable that Carrie, like Denise, would have had kids if she'd connected with a man who wanted to do so, and it's reasonable to assume that she would have enjoyed a life with children as much as the one she's created for herself without them.

QUESTIONS TO CONSIDER

What roles do cognitive dissonance and rationalization play in these adults' satisfaction with their childfree lives?

Why do you think some women feel ambivalent toward living childfree, while others are more confidently content with their situation?

Had they become parents, do you think these women would have expressed a similar level of satisfaction in that role as they have in their childfree status?

Childfree by Choice

"I do not want children. When I see children, I feel nothing. I have no maternal instinct. I am barren. I ovulate sand . . . I look at children and feel no pull toward them, no desire whatsoever. Actually, my fiancé and I have seen some very interesting personal ads of 50-year-olds that like to wear diapers. So we're thinking of adopting one of these guys. A baby by choice."

—Margaret Cho, comedian

Some people say that they've always known they didn't want to have children. For them, this is a *deliberate choice*. The National Center for Health Statistics reported that 6.6 percent of women of childbearing age indicated that they were *voluntarily childfree* in 1995, up from 4.3 percent in 1990.[2] Adults who say they've never wanted kids have some unique qualities not found in other categories of childfree adults. The intentionally childfree adults I met and interviewed for this book tended to be particularly independent and, by and large, to be living nontraditional lives.

A perfect example is Suzanne, a slim, athletic, thirty-seven-year-old, who is currently working as a legal secretary, but who's worked in male-dominated professions, such as construction and commercial fishing. She and her husband, John, have been together for fifteen years, and it's the first marriage for both of them. When I asked Suzanne how she ended up childfree, she shared, "I never had a strong inclination to be a mother, and up until my thirties, I was totally opposed to it. John has never wanted to have children, and he made this clear when we first met. I think that, had I really wanted to have a child, he might have eventually consented, but I feel strongly that unless both partners wholeheartedly want to have kids, they shouldn't have them." Suzanne recalled that there was only one short period of time when she questioned her decision. She explained, "I was thirty, and I'd been laid off from my construction job, a job I loved. I don't think the issue would have arisen had I still been completely absorbed in a fantastic, fulfilling career, but because I was unemployed and at a crossroads, I had enough time in my personal life to stop and thoroughly think things through. I spent several months examining the pros and cons and talking to my husband before feeling fully resigned to a life without children."

Suzanne was one of the few women I interviewed who talked about actually taking the time to fully process the final decision of whether or not to become a parent. According to a Guttmacher Institute survey, nearly 50 percent of pregnancies in the United States are unplanned.[3] Imagine living in a world in which every single individual of childbearing age took the time to mull over the decision about whether or not to have children, rather than simply allowing pregnancy to *happen*—how many *fewer* children would be conceived?

According to a Guttmacher Institute survey, over 50 percent of pregnancies in the United States are unplanned.

Suzanne shared the common sentiment that only when her friends began to have children did she begin to question herself. She wondered if it was a kind of midlife transition, explaining, "I've noticed that people who don't have children suddenly decide they're ready to do so in their mid-thirties. When I really examined my own options, though, I knew that having kids was not the right choice for my husband and me. I look at my brother, and how dependent he is on Mom, because he has a daughter and he's a single dad. I believe the level of involvement in my brother's life is a huge burden on our mother, and yet she seems to feel obligated to sacrifice her own independence to be supportive of her son and grandchild. Being a parent is a lifelong commitment."

Suzanne went on to say, "I feel strongly about experiencing life, so when I think about the fact that I will never carry a child in my womb and give birth, or share in my husband's love for our child,

I feel sad. Yet, this is still not enough of a reason to make me want to have children. The sacrifices that are required are just too great, and I know that I just don't have it in me to do it the way I imagine I would want to. In a weird sense, I feel that I'm sacrificing for the ultimate good of my unborn child."

Even though Suzanne expressed certainty about her decision and relayed that she has been clear for years that she didn't want to have kids, the emotional pain related to the absence of that experience in her life is very palpable. She expressed the same ambivalence described by adults who wanted children, but were unable to have them, whose stories are told later in this chapter. Suzanne's life with her husband is also similar to the lives of the Childfree by Happenstance, for whom having a child "just didn't happen," the difference being that she and her husband started their relationship with the intention to remain childfree while the other couples started out assuming that they would have kids someday. In Suzanne, we see a woman who has, from time to time, stepped back and questioned if she made the right choice. Most of us do this in our lives, whether it's with relationships, careers, or where we live. The questioning period is usually brief, and then we're back to feeling good about the choices we've made.

"Having kids is just not something I've ever been interested in. I don't think babies are cute. I don't like to hold them or be around them."

"I started with the *no kids* talk by the time I was about twelve years old," relayed Laurie, a forty-three-year-old engineer, who is married to her high school sweetheart Craig, a mechanic. "It's just not something I've ever been interested in. I don't think babies are cute. I don't like to hold them or be around them. Toddlers are barely tolerable to me. Kids start to be considered real people in my book around age ten or so. I was fortunate enough to find a man with the same opinion of kids, so we were on the same page regarding children from the beginning. We are very happy with our decision not to have kids. One of the factors is that we're both pretty selfish with our time, toys, and money. We share it all with each other, but don't want to split any of that up with kids. Craig and I enjoy spending a lot of time together and doing things spontaneously. It's a very rewarding and fun-filled lifestyle."

Nicole, a thirty-seven-year-old FBI agent who lives with her three large dogs in her home outside of Washington DC, is equally adamant about never having wanted children. Nicole insisted, "Even when I was a child in elementary school, kids always seemed like more of a burden to their parents than anything else. When I was eleven, my mom had a baby, and I spent my teenage years as the unpaid live-in babysitter, which basically sealed the deal on my decision to not have children."

Nicole's childhood was painful for her, and this probably resulted in her closing the door on the possibility that she might want to be a mother. She was not willing to consider that raising children might be a pleasurable experience for both parent and child.

Arno, a retired respiratory therapist, age sixty, laughed when he told me, "I've never had anyone ask me about my experience of not having children. I never thought about it at all until about two years ago. Reading through your interview questions made me feel sad for a few days, but now I mostly feel relief. My wife and I helped to raise our best friend's child, William, and he was the sweetest boy. Then when he turned sixteen, he turned into a horrible person. I'm kind of relieved that I didn't have to go through that. We have lots of friends whose children have grown up and are honest and industrious, but for whatever reason, William got into drugs and crime. I married a woman who couldn't have kids. We got together when I was thirty, and I didn't really think about it at the time. Then, by the time I did think about it, I was fifty-eight and it was too late." Arno went on to say, "I firmly believe that in the next one hundred years the earth is going to become a very unpleasant place. I've always felt this way, though, filled with gloom and doom. Humans have made a mess of things, and every day they prove how much more of a mess we are willing to make of it. Parents are too busy to contemplate it. Humans almost always choose the irresponsible shortcut rather than acting responsibly!"

I asked Arno what triggered his thoughts of being a dad when he was in his late fifties, but he had no answer for me. I suppose it could have been his observation of the children in his life growing into young adults, some doing well while others were struggling, and possibly imagining what kind of young adult kids he may have had at that point in life. As a man, he had the luxury of not being exposed to the same societal and family pressures to have children that many women describe.

Jill, a forty-three-year-old network engineer, is childfree mostly by design but also somewhat by default. She heard about my project from a friend, and we met at the end of her workday at my office. "I don't think that you and I would be talking had I not been lucky as an adolescent. I had a boyfriend in high school and I was naïve about contraception. It was just by chance that I didn't become pregnant. I guess I always assumed that I'd have kids until I became aware that I had a choice about it. I went from undergraduate to graduate school and one of my professors, who was about forty, didn't have kids. She was a public health nurse. She was the first woman I had known who consciously didn't have children. I thought about it, and I couldn't think of anyone who had made that conscious choice—all the women I knew who didn't have kids were unable to have them. Because I met this woman when I was twenty-four, at an age when I was making decisions about my life, the assumption that I would have children simply disappeared. I never revisited it. There has been a total of about half an hour when I've thought about it through all these years." Jill added that she and her partner of five years, Susan, have at times joked about having a child of their own. Susan has one grown daughter, who she raised mostly on her own. Jill shared, "We took care of Susan's three-year-old nephew recently for a few days. I had a great time with him, but I was exhausted by the time he left. Thank God we could tag-team for those three days. Susan was much less patient than me—after he left, she turned to me laughing and said, 'This seals it. Now I know I'm done!'"

In Jill's case, it was her chance meeting of just one individual that planted the seed of the idea that not having children was an actual possibility. As more adults choose the childfree path, the impact on the younger generation will no doubt be enormous. I have experienced this when talking through the possibility of not having children with younger women versus older women. When I bring it up with women in their twenties, I can almost see the wheels begin to turn in their minds as they realize that this is yet another big life choice that is placed in their hands to make—having children doesn't have to be a given.

Tracy is a forty-seven-year-old self-employed web designer who works from home and spends, by her own estimation, 90 percent of her time alone. She was eager to talk about her experiences being childfree, sharing, "I feel very clear about my decision. I've never had any motherhood instinct. When I was thirty-two or thirty-three, I did a casual survey of my friends who have kids, five or six families. They all said that they never knew it would take so much time. After that I felt complete, especially because I didn't have a partner with whom I wanted to have children. I was sure about my decision because of having taken the time to talk to my friends with kids." She added, "I have no regrets at all. My parents never even asked me about it or about my not getting married. They were very good about it, and this is something I should thank them for."

Like Suzanne, the legal secretary, Tracy described feeling quite certain of her choice but then wanting to confirm it by doing a little field research. Having parents who did not put pressure on her to marry or to have children certainly contributed to her being able to give herself permission to choose the life path that she truly wanted for herself.

Mark and Sarah, a professional couple in their mid-fifties who live in Portland, Oregon, have been married for six years. Mark shared, "I was married before, at age twenty-six. My wife and I were not enthusiastic about the institution of marriage, nor were we interested in making a family. At the time, we felt the traditional concepts of American life were deeply flawed, but we got married because I could get my wife benefits through work. Then we went willingly along the career path, me for security, my wife more out of ambition. In many ways we wanted to avoid family ties, and we saw having children as a kind of trap. We talked it over from time to time during those first ten years, and we decided not to have kids. After twenty-four years of marriage, we divorced. My ex-wife remarried, to a widower with two college-aged daughters, and I've been told that she has very much enjoyed taking on a mother role with them." Sarah's marriage to Mark was her first, at age forty-nine. She shared, "As a girl, I assumed I would marry and have children and I looked forward to my role as a mother; the right opportunity never materialized and I didn't want to be a single parent. I have a close family and this gives Mark and me the opportunity to provide a great deal of love, care, and support to my nieces and nephews. In many ways, we've shared parenting with my sisters."

"I've never, ever, had a baby urge," insisted Annie, a thirty-five-year-old vocational counselor married to Roger, a thirty-eight-year-old financial analyst. "We both came into the relationship knowing that we didn't want children, so we never really talked about it. In my last relationship it was a huge issue—it finally became the deal breaker for us! My boyfriend wanted to have children, and I didn't think that I did. I went to see a counselor to talk about it, and for a couple of years there I tried to spend as much time as I could around kids. I also talked to lots of people with and without children. This process validated my sense that having kids wasn't the right choice for me, and so I broke off the relationship. I recently had to have my tubes tied for medical reasons, and so I had six weeks to think it through again once and for all. I went away for a weekend with a couple of my girlfriends and their babies and this reinforced my decision to be childfree." Roger shared, "I feel like I've been thinking about it for a long time. In my previous marriage, we decided early on not to have kids. Despite this, I reached a point of looking at friends with children and realizing that I was passing a certain window of opportunity. I had to ask myself if this was something I wanted to get in on as well, but it just didn't seem appealing to me. I've often thought that if I were in a financial position to have kids with a full-time nanny, I might do so, or if I could guarantee that my children would be emotionally and physically healthy and that they would be there for me in my old age. Of course, you can't guarantee this, and I'm not willing to take the risk." Annie added, "Having kids would introduce a chaotic element into our lives that I wouldn't be able to control, and this is a huge issue that reinforces my decision. I watch my friends with children and see the struggles they have in their relationships. Plus, I see that they are always tired and so I know that having kids would take a toll on my health."

Their story reminded me of Nicole, the FBI agent who knew as a teenager that she didn't want to have kids. Annie and Roger have a similar cautious and protective perspective of life, and choosing to close the door on having kids feels safer than having them and not being able to predict if the experience would be enjoyable or not.

QUESTIONS TO CONSIDER

Do men and women who have always known that they didn't want to have kids have greater need for control and certainty than others?

In what ways are men treated differently than women in our culture with regard to their choice to have kids or not?

Is this changing over time?

Do lesbians feel less societal pressure to become mothers than other women?

Childfree by Circumstance

> *"'No, no, sorry. I don't have any . . .' Why does this always*
> *seem to be the first thing I'm asked? It takes my breath away,*
> *yet why do I feel the need to apologize for my reply? Look-*
> *ing vague and embarrassed, my questioner glances over my*
> *shoulder for someone else to talk to: someone with whom he*
> *or she has more in common, someone with children."*
>
> —Nancy Rome, writer for the *Washington Post*

Some childfree adults have yearned for a baby but have been unable to make it happen due to infertility or other factors. Writer Nancy Rome wrote an article about her own experience of delivering a stillborn baby and the impact of being constantly asked if she has children. She refers to herself as "childless" and has emotional pain related to not having had children. I'd argue that part of her pain stems from our national obsession with motherhood. Every time I get online, there's a story about some Hollywood celebrity getting pregnant or having a baby. Several television programs glorify the lives of large families. It's become an obsession in our culture. When I see the stories of Hollywood pregnancies I feel like an outlier, an anomaly, because I am not a mother. Likewise, when I see the programs depicting large, happy families, it makes me feel like I may have missed out on an exciting and rich life experience. It's a subtle message that having children and large families is not only the norm, but also something to be celebrated and praised. For an individual or couples who truly want to have children, but are unable to do so, these media displays must be exceedingly painful to see.

Many childless adults try to find a way to accept their situation and to build a rich and full life for themselves without kids. A good example of this is Renee, a university librarian in her early sixties. She got married the first time when she was just eighteen years old. "I was married very young to my college boyfriend. The marriage was a mistake, the circumstance being that I got pregnant. I had a miscarriage between our engagement announcement and the proposed wedding date. We kept the wedding date, probably at my insistence, and then moved to Nashville for my husband to go to graduate school. I worked while he went to school. At that time, all kinds of social norms were being broken down, in large part because of the Pill. Although we were married, we 'explored' other relationships, with at least some knowledge on the part of each other. Our marriage wasn't a relationship either of us had the slightest interest of bringing children into. When the marriage ended, I put myself through graduate school, and I settled into my career. I met my second husband, David, and this marriage turned out to be everything my first was not. David was older than me, and he had three children from his prior marriage who were with us from time to time. We agreed that having children of our own would not be the best thing for us. David didn't feel that he could raise a second family, and I thought it would be more unfair to ask this of him than it would be for me to remain childless. Despite this, I did become pregnant in my late thirties, and David and I decided that having an abortion was the best decision for us. At the time, it seemed the right thing to do, but over the next few

> "I became pregnant in my late thirties, and David and I decided that having an abortion was the best decision for us. At the time, it seemed the right thing to do, but over the next few years and then decades, it became one of the most painful realities of my life."

years and then decades, it became one of the most painful realities of my life."

For Renee, being childfree was just a circumstance of her life until she became pregnant and had an abortion. This choice forced her to come face to face with the reality that maybe she would have liked to have had a child of her own. She expressed regrets and quite a lot of grief about her decision. Had she had the child, he or she would now be a young adult, and I could see that Renee still struggles with the loss of what might have been.

Miriam, an eighty-nine-year-old divorcée and retired university administrator, is another childless woman who has grieved over her inability to have children. Miriam shared, "I think my circumstances are a little different from most other childless women. I feel very deprived about it. My uncle raped me when I was twelve, and he gave me a venereal disease that resulted in sterility. I have always felt inferior to other women because of not being able to have children. Even now, I can be in the grocery store and I'll see a baby and she and I will get into an eye lock—sometimes I'll wave and the baby will wave back. The mother won't even know. The baby makes such a quick connection, and it's a magical moment for me. Sometimes the connection feels quite intense. I've had to accept that this is all I get of my wish to have a baby. In all these years, I've never lost the wish to have children, never." Miriam shared that she is continually reminded of her rape and of being unable to become pregnant. "I've never forgotten that incident—it's a vivid replay of a film that comes back to me in Technicolor at least once a week." She also had the expectation, even after her divorce in 1960, that if she met a man and fell in love, she would tell him about her infertility and he would reject her. In her marriage, she tried to convince her husband to consider adoption—there was a child in their life that they might have been able to adopt—but her husband had no interest in raising children. Although she had siblings, she had no nieces or nephews.

Miriam has never been able to feel a sense of peace with not being a mom because she is unable to use healthy defensive coping tools such as rationalization. As children, we learn these defenses from our parents; Miriam's father was not a part of her life and her mother was emotionally absent. She never healed from her rape, and I would guess that she never told her mother about the incident. Details were not discussed and nurturing and support were not available. Miriam went on to choose a spouse who was not nurturing and was unwilling to work together with her on making life decisions. Furthermore, through the years she aligned herself with a group of women who were mothers, rather than seeking out friends who, like her, did not have children, and thus she felt like an outsider. It's almost as if she felt the need to punish herself, which is often one of the tragic results of women who blame themselves for their sexual abuse. If she did not talk about it, she was unable to receive the comforting message that it was not her fault. In a sense, Miriam has used rationalization but in an unhealthy way: to explain why her life has been miserable.

"I had a client many years ago who'd had something go wrong physically in her early twenties and she was crazed about not being able to have kids. She always had a big empty hole, and she ended up killing herself. She could not deal with her inability to have children."

Trish, the divorced psychotherapist, shared with me the story of one of her patients whose life was tormented because of not having children. She related, "I had a client many years ago who'd had something go wrong physically in her early twenties and she was crazed about not being able to have kids. She always had a big empty hole, and she ended up killing herself. She could not deal with her inability to have children. I also recall a colleague, another therapist, who was emotionally pained every month when her period came along. Her husband wouldn't consider adoption."

Our individual psychological styles and worldviews impact how we cope with our life circumstances. Two individuals may have quite different responses to quite similar experiences. One person holds on to what they missed out on or the grief and pain associated with something from their past, while another person focuses on the future or even decides that what happened has impacted them in a positive way.

Are you:

Childfree by Happenstance

Childfree by Choice

Childfree by Circumstance

QUESTIONS TO CONSIDER

What personality characteristics have resulted in these women feeling such intense grief after so many years despite having had rich lives in many ways?

Why have they been unable to use the coping tool of rationalization in a healthy manner?

The Norm of Ambiguity

Reading through the stories of childfree adults, it's clear that emotion around this life decision is not cut and dried. There is confusion and second-guessing at times. For some, regret follows years of relative peace around the decision, while others experience peace after years of uncertainty or grief. Many individuals may find themselves identifying with each of the three categories of childfree adults at various points in their lives—this is normal and a reflection of the ambiguity of living. The critical issue is being aware of our inner processes and having the ability to manage negative emotion and confusion when it arises. These topics are explored more fully in chapter 2.

QUESTIONS TO CONSIDER

Are you childfree because it just didn't happen, because of choice, or because you were unable to have children?

Do you, in some ways, fit into each of the three categories of childfree adults?

Even if you're at peace with your decision to not have kids, are there times when you feel a loss because of pressures from friends and family or from the media?

Have you noticed cognitive dissonance or rationalization in yourself?

When you rationalize, do you do so in a healthy or an unhealthy way?

Whose stories are you most able to relate to?

CHAPTER 2
CHILDFREE DECISION MAKING: A BEHIND-THE-SCENES LOOK

"Too many people spend money they haven't earned, to buy things they don't want, to impress people they don't like."
—Will Rogers

Life is filled with opportunities to choose, but in many instances, where we end up seems to be mostly thanks to chance or luck. In chapter 1, a variety of adults described the various pathways they took in arriving at a childfree status. Most of these individuals reported feeling good about the place they were in life, but others felt a sense of uncertainty because they thought they may have missed out or made the wrong choice. It's not uncommon, even when we are happy with a particular decision, to occasionally wonder if it was right for us. Our individual personalities and certain psychological processes impact the way we make decisions, interpret situations, and handle ambiguity. Taking time to explore in depth the factors that influenced our life paths leads to increased clarity about why our lives turned out as they did. This facilitates acceptance of—and insight into—ways to improve our current situation.

Kids—To Have or Not to Have

Having the opportunity to decide whether or not to have children is a fairly new phenomenon brought about by the introduction of the Pill in the 1960s. Even now, decades later, most young adults still assume that they will have kids, simply because this continues to be the norm in our society. There does, however, appear to be a growing movement toward not having kids. In Japan and Western Europe, there has been a decline in birthrate, a trend that's catching on here in North America despite the glamorization of large families by the media.

In the not-too-distant past, most adults didn't make a decision about whether or not to have children. My friend Karen recalls sitting in a zoology class in college in 1959 and listening to a lecture about human reproduction. Her professor shared with the class of eighteen-year-olds that there was a new pill that could keep women from getting pregnant. The FDA approved the marketing of these oral contraceptive pills on May 9, 1960. By the time I went to college, eighteen years later, the Pill was a primary form of birth control, available in college campus health clinics and considered to be safe and effective. Even then, however, we didn't openly discuss whether or not we wanted to be parents the way we talked about our choices of careers or where we hoped to live after graduating from college. The assumption was that we would get married and have families of our own, the way our parents did. And this is still the norm. Providers of premarital counseling, such as churches and couple's counselors, don't routinely ask couples whether or not they want to have children, because the assumption is made that people will simply have kids. When the subject of children comes up, it's usually focused on differences in child-rearing styles, rather than whether or not the couple actually wants to have kids.

Many folks who reached adulthood prior to the Pill's widespread availability, or who stepped into the role of being a parent

Having the opportunity to decide whether or not to have children is a fairly new phenomenon brought about by the introduction of the Pill in the 1960s.

without giving it a second thought, recognize that having children might have been something they would have gone into with a little more discernment given the opportunity. Recently, we invited some neighbors, two couples in their late sixties and seventies, over for dinner. Given that this topic was front and center in my life as I wrote this book, we began to discuss the fact that more women are opting out of parenthood. Doris, who is in her mid-seventies and has been with her husband since high school, became quite emotional, and exclaimed, "We didn't have a choice about it! I was expected to just get married and to then have a family. That was what people did. If you didn't have children, it was because you weren't physically able to do so." Doris has a daughter in her mid-forties who has no children. I've never once heard Doris express sadness about her daughter having missed out because of not having kids; instead, she talks with pride about the career path her daughter has taken and the freedom that she and her husband have in their mid-life. After Doris's emotional outcry, my other neighbor shared the story of her friend who has recently begun to lament having children because of the estranged relationship that she has with her adult son.

Three shifts in our society are happening simultaneously—the availability of a choice of whether or not to have children, the acceptance of not having children, and the willingness on the part of some parents to acknowledge disappointment in their kids. Susan Jeffers's book *I'm*

> "We didn't have a choice about it! I was expected to just get married and to then have a family. That was what people did. If you didn't have children, it was because you weren't physically able to do so."

> Three Societal Shifts: The choice of whether or not to have children. The acceptance of not having children. The willingness on the part of some parents to acknowledge disappointment in their children.

Okay, You're a Brat! Setting the Priorities Straight and Freeing You from the Guilt and Mad Myths of Parenthood gives an inside look at the not-so-pleasant side of parenting and challenges readers who don't already have children to face the reality of what parenting is all about. Jeffers emphasizes the difference between loving your children and actually enjoying parenting them. One reader wrote, "After reading Dr. Jeffers's book, I was relieved to know that having mixed feelings about parenting is normal, and that there are many sacrifices and unpleasant times associated with parenting. The thing I regret most is that everyone told me how amazingly fulfilling and fun mothering is, without mentioning the negatives, and especially the fact that once you sign on for the job you cannot quit." Readers of books on the struggles of parenting include not only parents needing validation that their struggles and mixed feelings about child rearing are normal, but also young people who are still trying to decide whether or not they want to have children.

QUESTIONS TO CONSIDER

What was the primary birth control method used at the time you reached your childbearing years?

Have you heard older parents talk about their own lack of choice?

How have your own parents reacted to your thoughts about not having children?

Have you had friends who were able to talk about their disappointments in parenting?

Decision Making

As I discussed in chapter 1, chance factors in my life rather than deliberate decision making resulted in my not being a mom. But because I never really made a conscious decision on the matter, I lacked a sense of closure around it until I was well into my forties. Looking back, I can see that the availability of reliable and convenient birth control certainly played a role here; this allowed me to hold off on thinking about children until I was ready to do so. This day didn't come until it was practically too late to choose a different path. At that point, in my mid-forties, I suddenly realized that the door was almost closed on the chance to have a child of my own. This realization was triggered by my getting involved with a man who had children, causing me to wonder if I was missing out on a necessary life experience. I had a lot of confusion during this time because my logical self knew that I had already made the decision and felt good about it, but my emotional self kept interrupting and saying, "Hey, you might have made a mistake. If you hurry, you could still have a child!" I wanted to have a sense of closure and peace with this decision, and the approach I took in attaining this was to explore all the reasons that people have kids, including the positives and negatives of being a parent. I did this in a typical decision-making manner, almost as if I were thirty and looking ahead. I believed that this exploration would either tell me that I would make the same decision if I had it to do over again, or it would lead me to take the steps to bring a child into my life. I actually felt some trepidation about delving into it, because I feared doing so would cause emotional pain. Also, if I were to ultimately decide that I really did want to have a baby, the result would be life changing.

Babylust

My first step was to examine all the reasons people have children and to recognize which factors were pushing me at that particular time in my life, my mid-forties, when the window of opportunity for having a child was quickly coming to a close. The most obvious, of course, is the yearning for a baby that some people describe as a biological urge. A colleague of mine shared that she often sees couples in her practice who are in conflict over whether or not to have a child. In fact, she recently witnessed two female patients leave their fiancés after the men announced that they did not want to have children. The desire that these two women felt to have children was stronger than their desire to stay with the men they loved. I simply could not relate to this experience. As I shared in chapter 1, the men in my life have not wanted to have children, but I never once considered leaving a relationship because of this, even if I felt having a baby was what I truly wanted to do.

My experience of feeling so nonchalant about being a mother throughout most of my adult life is dramatically different from the "babylust" I hear others describe. When I met with Miriam, the eighty-nine-year-old woman who still grieves not having been able to have children, she told me about her lifelong yearning to be a mother. "I remember when I had my first period, understanding that I was becoming a woman. I was reading a magazine and discovered a series of photographs of children taken by a famous photographer. I cut those pictures out and taped them up on the wall around my bed. Even then, at twelve years of age, I was crazy about babies, and for all these years, my attraction to children has never ended." Miriam's strong desire to have a child of her own and her inability to do so resulted in an unmet need that simply grew over time. She told me that she looked at other women who were mothers and envied their lives. She also felt "less-than" because of her inability to conceive. Her babylust began while she was still a child herself and apparently never waned.

Two of the women I interviewed are happily single and are childfree by happenstance, as they assumed they'd settle down and have families of their own, but this never came to pass. They shared that they have never experienced a strong maternal urge. Denise, the psychiatric office manager, noted, "I do believe that people can have an irresistible longing to have a child or children, but whether this is innate, societal, or peer driven is unclear to me. I have a feeling it may be a bit of all three." Jackie, the paralegal who has never been married, also reported never having had a yearning for a child of her own. I guessed that these women may have not experienced a strong maternal urge because of the lack of an appropriate partner with whom to raise a child. If their situations had been different, they'd likely have become mothers, because growing up, both always assumed they would have families of their own. Through the years, Jackie and Denise no doubt suppressed any maternal urges that were triggered by situational factors—such as scenes in movies or observing parents in loving interactions with their children— and doing so was, for them, a healthy response. Denise told me that early on, she really wanted to be a mother, but because her husband was mentally ill and therefore unstable, she decided that having children with him would be unwise. She seems to have accepted this as the way things were meant to be and has not fought to change her destiny. After her divorce in her late thirties, she did not seek out other partners with whom to have children; she viewed the window of opportunity for childbearing as having passed. However, Denise never had an extremely strong maternal drive. Adults who, on the other hand, wanted very much to have children but kept being blocked by life circumstances such as infertility, are more likely to focus intently on what they have missed out on and to experience a keen sense of grief and loss as a result.

It's common for childfree adults to assert not having strong maternal or paternal urges. When I asked Carrie, the fifty-one-year-old medical biller also childfree by happenstance, if she ever felt the ticking of her biological clock, she replied, "I never experienced it. I never had a yearning. That's what I was waiting for. If I'd had that feeling, I'd have acted on it." Chris and I were out at a restaurant recently when we ran into a couple we know. They were out to dinner with their daughter, son-in-law, and infant granddaughter. The woman said, "Ellen, you've got to meet Susanna," and she brought the baby, who was sleeping, over to our table. I didn't know how to respond, but I was certain that I didn't want to hold the child. I

"I never experienced it. I never had a yearning. That's what I was waiting for. If I'd had that feeling, I'd have acted on it."

made a few ooh and aah sounds before she whisked Susanna away. I can recall having this exact same experience way back in my twenties, when I went with my friend to visit her brother, who had a newborn baby. If I hadn't been so focused at the time on traveling and on plans for graduate school, perhaps I would have been more interested in the baby my friend was encouraging me to hold. My recollection, though, is that my response to the baby was different from that of my friend, who was also busy with traveling and pursuing higher education, but who seemed to cherish the opportunity to hold this small child. Through the years, my response has been consistent, and at some point I began to experience an actual sense of distaste around many small children, noticing that they make a lot of noise, demand attention, and often have sticky fingers and drool running down their little chins. I've not been around kids enough to experience the positives of them, and to experience how these may outweigh the unpleasant attributes. It's reasonable to assert that some people are baby people and others are not, just as some people are dog people or cat people while others are not. Since early childhood, I've fit into the animal person category.

After twenty-five years of owning cats I went through several years of not having pets, but as I approached forty, I began to have a strong desire to nurture someone or something. I certainly wouldn't describe this as babylust, which I experienced only briefly in my mid-forties, because my response to the yearning was exploring options and ultimately adopting a small, black terrier named Bella. She was adorable, and I bonded with her instantly. Bella was the perfect solution and fulfilled my need to nurture. I have been surprised with my patience for Bella and with the sacrifices I've been willing to make to ensure that she feels safe and loved. Caring for a dog has provided plenty of unconditional love and just enough responsibility—much less responsibility than a child would require. Having Bella has not interfered with my career or put a dent in my finances. For me, this has been a perfect fit. There have been days when I've felt overwhelmed by the level of commitment it takes to be "mother" to a dog, and during these times, I've had a sense of relief to not have the much greater responsibility of being mother to a child. My dog is very much like a child to me, and I find that other childfree adults view their pets in the same way. One patient, Sandra, sends out photos of her Dalmatian to friends and relatives with the same frequency as any parent. She takes her dog to day care and hires in-home sitters when she goes out of town. Many childfree adults, including myself, display their pets' pictures at work. Cara Swann, a writer for Suite101, interviewed a woman who shared, "My desk is covered with pictures of my pets. I always point them out to those who inquire that they are my family and that I don't have or want human kids. I've had a couple of people react negatively, but by and large, I've gotten neutral or positive feedback."[4] I have had parents of children argue that the love for a pet cannot match the love for a child, and I cannot understand why they feel the need to challenge this. An Associated Press–Petside. com poll found half of all American pet owners consider their pets as much a part of the family as any person in the household.[5] It was helpful for me to realize that others feel as bonded to their pets as I do to my dog. She meets a need that I have, the desire to form a secure attachment to another living being. It is irrelevant to argue about whether my love for her is as strong as the love a parent feels for a child—the critical issue is my recognition of this need and the realization that I've found the best way for me to fulfill this need.

The Biological Clock

Another factor that pushed me to consider having a child was the last-minute realization, in my mid-forties, that I had one last chance to jump aboard the parent train. The biological clock ticks because the optimal time for having a child is passing; for most of us this is sometime in our thirties or forties. Allowing that time frame to pass brings challenges and awkwardness as we experience our peers, one by one, beginning to have children. I asked other childfree adults, both childfree by choice and by happenstance, whether

Some Negative Reasons People Have Children:
- **Babylust**
- **The Biological Clock**
- **Pressure from Media, Family, and Friends**
- **Fear of Missing Out**
- **Proving Our Parenting Skills**
- **Avoiding Being Mislabeled or Misunderstood**
- **Idealization of Child Rearing**

they'd experienced this kind of biological clock sensation: the realization that their child-bearing opportunities were coming to an end. When I spoke with Suzanne, the thirty-seven-year-old legal secretary who is childfree by choice, she shared, "I think it's possible that my biological clock period may have coincided with my career change because I found myself with time on my hands and at a starting-over point in my life. I also think the need to address the kid issue had to do with people in our social circle starting families and my need to be okay with *not* having kids. Even if I didn't want children, I still needed to know that I had thought it through, talked about everything with my husband, and made a definitive decision."

Suzanne implies here that she might not have felt any kind of internal clock ticking if it weren't for her career change and pressure from her friends. She might not even have contemplated whether or not she wanted to have kids. Observing the lives of others is often the catalyst that nudges me into thinking about my own choices. It's reminiscent of the feeling I sometimes get when I drive by a runner and think, *If I want to run a marathon, I'd better do so before I get any older.* But later, when I sit down and contemplate the training schedule, I usually decide that it's not the right choice for me, and I can

"I have a friend who said that her womb ached after she'd been married for a year and she and her husband hadn't started moving towards having kids."

let that particular life experience go. Of course, the experience of child rearing carries a whole different dimension of meaning in a person's life than running a marathon. But the point is I might not even be tempted by the idea of one if it weren't for the passing thought I have when I see a runner pushing herself when I'm out doing my daily errands.

Jill, the network engineer who, like Suzanne, is childfree by choice, shared, "I've never felt the ticking of a biological clock, and none of the women I've been involved with ever wanted to have kids. I've been with Susan for five years now, and this is the first time I've been with a partner who has a child. Susan's daughter is in her mid-twenties, and I like being a part of her life. I don't think gay and lesbian couples have the same societal expectation to have children, and making it happen takes planning, obviously. When a gay couple has a child it's because they really want to do so, not because they don't want to feel left out or because of accidental pregnancy."

Without the same peer pressure, gays and lesbians are able to make a clearer decision about kids. In some arenas they may even be pressured to not have children. Gays and lesbians who do decide to have children get the opportunity to soul search in a way that other couples don't, as they must have an intense desire to parent since there is so much involved in either getting pregnant or finding a surrogate or choosing to adopt. This same principal applies to couples who struggle with infertility. Elizabeth is a forty-eight-year-old marketing consultant from Massachusetts who has also known since early adulthood that she did not want to have children. She and her partner, Maria, have been together for several years now and they, like me, have a small dog who meets their needs for nurturing. Elizabeth shared, "When I was forty-two, I experienced the ticking of my biological clock and got wound up for a brief moment. This feeling came back when I reached the age of forty-five, because I had a sense of knowing that my time was running out, and I felt sad about this. I was, however, very secure in myself, happy with my life, and I didn't feel the need or desire for children. If I'd truly wanted a child, I would have adopted. I think my sadness was just my realization that I was getting older." Elizabeth's observation brings out a different issue entirely, that at certain times in our lives we become aware of our own mortality—one way to ensure that we live on is through having children. Children, in a sense, connect us to the future.

Annie and Roger, a couple in their mid-thirties who are child-free by choice, described their thoughts on the biological clock phenomenon. Annie, a vocational counselor, shared, "I definitely believe in the biological clock, because for years I'd go out to breakfast with my friends and they'd see a baby in the restaurant and go crazy!" Her husband Roger agreed, noting, "I have a friend who said that her womb ached after she'd been married for a year and she and her husband hadn't started moving towards having kids." He paused, collecting his thoughts before continuing, "It's hard, though, to separate the biological from what we think. There are moments when I'm feeling fond about children and I think it would be nice to have a little version of myself. This usually happens when I'm around a friend and his or her child and they're having a close, bonding experience with one another." Annie jumped in to share, "My experience is just the opposite, since Mom wasn't around and I had to do so much child rearing for my sister. It was really hard, and I felt like I got all the bad aspects of parenting without any of the rewarding ones." Annie's experience of being the caretaker for her sister and not feeling nurtured by her mother is a clear example of a reason why someone would move into adulthood and not feel a strong urge to have a child. She never had that illusory glow about being a mom that is common for so many young women. Roger, on the other hand, seems to have entered adulthood with more of a neutral perception of parenting, which has resulted in him swaying emotionally back and forth depending on which children he is around.

Men's biological clocks may look different from women's simply because they are capable of producing children at any age. Arno, the retired respiratory therapist, hadn't experienced a biological clock until two years ago, at age fifty-eight. He stated, "I believe in the biological clock. You just wake up one morning when the alarm goes off. I realized one day that I would never have kids, that my name would die with me, and it's kind of a shame."

Where the biological clock phenomenon is concerned, it's clear that more than a pure desire to be a parent is involved. Part of it is classic peer pressure—watching your friends start to have kids and realizing that you're going to be left out of the group is a strong factor. The other part is chance—who you end up with romantically and what activities you're involved in serve to fill up your time and expend your emotional energy. But regardless of why it occurs, for those who experience it, the biological clock feels very real.

Pressure from Media, Family, and Friends

Plenty of people have kids because of cultural pressure, much of which comes from our media. In the mid-1980s, there was a popular song about a woman who thought she had it all until she became a mother, and then she realized what life was really all about. I recall being offended by this message, with its implication that a woman's place is in the home changing diapers rather than out in the world competing with men. The song even insinuates that it's selfish for a woman to choose to be childfree. Annie, the vocational counselor, mused, "People have often said to me that having children is a great way to give back and to contribute to society. I realized that I was already doing that through my job. I feel that there's a certain judgment around not having kids; people just assume that you'll do it, and when you don't, you're viewed as strange."

Jill, the network engineer, shared, "I have a lot of friends now who don't have kids; most of them are in their late thirties or early forties. Most of my lesbian friends don't have children, and most of my straight friends do. Gay women don't have the same pressure to produce. My friend, Morgan, had a bridal shower recently, and the women there began to ask her when she was going to have kids. They even played a game predicting how many children she would have. I used to be involved with a Lutheran church, and one fall I attended a women's retreat. At the retreat we were asked to go around, give our name, and tell how many children/grandchildren we had. I was the only one there, other than a Japanese exchange student, out of fifty women, who didn't have kids."

I can imagine how left out Jill must have felt at the retreat because I've experienced similar situations. I wouldn't be surprised if the Japanese student was influenced by the experience and became a mother, so that when she was Jill's age she wouldn't find herself in a room of other women feeling like an odd duck.

Some people are okay with being different from the norm.

Laurie, the forty-three-year-old engineer who has known since childhood that she didn't want to have kids, shared, "The expectation in our society is that after you've dated for some magical time period, you will get married, and the marriage will be followed by having children. Each person and each couple is unique in their desires and goals in life. Being married or reproducing is not nearly as important as having a happy, healthy relationship with a person you truly love and respect. I see some people getting these priorities turned around." During our telephone interview, I asked Laurie if her parents had an influence on her ability to be herself and not just follow the pack. She shared that she received tremendous support from home; her parents always attended her sports activities and allowed her to make choices about what activities she wanted to participate in. She claims that in the twenty years she's been with Craig, they have never felt any pressure from her parents to produce a grandchild.

Others do, however, feel pressure from family and friends to reproduce, and this pressure is often far from subtle. Sheila, the owner of a small bookstore, shared, "Back in the 1970s, when I was about thirty, shortly after Walt and I married, I attended a family reunion. My aunt ran across the room to me and asked when I was going to get pregnant. She told me that if I missed out on having a child, I'd regret it every single day for the rest of my life. I've thought about this so many times during the years, and I'm still waiting for that feeling of regret. It's simply never come!" Annie, the vocational counselor in her mid-thirties, had a similar experience. "When I broke up with my boyfriend, basically because he wanted children and I did not, it was kind of like coming out of the closet because I shared with my family what was going on. Accepting the fact that I would never have kids was a huge disappointment for my parents." This resonates with me because though my own parents never pressured me to have children, I know that they would have loved to be grandparents to a child of mine. When my father read one of the first sample chapters of this book, he told me how sad it made him feel. Deep down, I believe that he thought someday I'd call with the news that I was having a baby—this work symbolized the reality that it would never happen.

As with all choices in life, there is loss; in the case of being childfree, it's not having the grandparenting experience with your own parents. Grandparenting is yet another area in which there is huge societal pressure, with T-shirts and bumper stickers proclaiming the pride and joy in being a grandparent. As childfree adults reach the time in life when their own peers begin to become grandparents, there will be yet another period of loss and sense of awkwardness as the wallets are pulled out and photographs of the grandkids are passed around. It is especially important for childfree adults who very much wanted, but were unable to have, children to address their grief and to create comfortable social networks for themselves—otherwise they will continue to feel the pain of these losses long past their child-rearing years. Some may choose to surround themselves with childfree adults, while others will become closely involved with families and friends who have children.

Missing Out

The notion that men and women might "miss out" on the experience of raising a child is a widespread cautionary message. Among my peers almost everyone has children, and so I often hear about what an important and wonderful part of life being a parent is. In her memoir, *Waiting for Daisy: The True Story of One Couple's Quest to Have a Baby* (Bloomsbury Publishing, 2008), Peggy Orenstein describes how her husband-to-be talks about his desire to have a family. He compares life to an amusement park, saying that he wants to ride every ride at least once. He adds that having kids is like the big, scary roller coaster; if you skip the roller coaster, you'll still have fun, but you will have missed a significant part of the experience. The reality is that we cannot do everything that life has to offer; we have to make choices about which experiences are the most critical for us, and we have to feel okay about the ones we pass up.

The idea that we will miss out by not having kids is perpetuated by the insistence of many parents that raising children has been the *most* rewarding job of their entire lives. In my experience, parents aren't hesitant to share this, even with friends who don't have children. I'm typically able to hear this kind of remark and not feel that my life has been insignificant or that I've missed out on something essential, but at times these sentiments have caused me to feel momentary regret about not having kids. Parents who make these kinds of casual remarks probably have no idea of their effects on young adults who are still in the decision-making phase. Adults who are still contemplating whether or not to have kids often hear about what they will miss out on if they *don't* have children. When, if ever, does anyone talk to them about the kind of sacrifices they will have to make if they *do* have children?

> "My advice to anyone considering starting a family is to think about it and talk about it and then think about it and talk about it some more."

Proving Our Parenting Skills

Some people might be tempted to have a child to demonstrate that they can do it. The thought of wanting to prove my mothering skills popped up recently when I was talking to my friend Doug, age ninety-one. He said, "My advice to anyone considering starting a family is to think about it and talk about it and then think about it and talk about it some more." Doug then suggested that since I have been so successful in my career, and since I don't have children, it probably means that I would not have been a good mother. I felt hurt by his comment and even said that I disagreed, that I thought I would have been an excellent mom.

Avoiding Being Labeled or Misunderstood

Childfree adults are often mistakenly viewed as people who don't like children or who would have made lousy parents. Writer Polly Vernon wrote an article on the choice of whether or not to have kids for *The Observer* in February 2009, in which she proclaimed, "It takes guts to say you don't want children."[6] After the piece was published, she was lambasted by angry readers. In her June 14, 2009, *Observer* column, she wrote, "The reaction to the piece was terrifying. Emails and letters arrived, condemning me, expressing disgust. I was denounced as bitter, selfish, un-sisterly, unnatural, evil. I'm now routinely referred to as 'baby-hating journalist Polly Vernon.'"[7] It's hard to understand why some parents are so defensive when a childfree adult shares that he or she feels good about this life status. When this has happened to me recently, I've responded by saying that I'm not criticizing a person's choice to be a parent, but simply offering up the idea that parenting ought to be an option rather than an obligation and that just because a person doesn't have children, he or she does not necessarily dislike kids.

"It takes guts to say you don't want children."

Idealization of Child Rearing

Even for those childfree adults who know that not having kids was the best choice, there are times for most when they imagine how parenting might be a wonderful experience. For some, this tug comes as a result of a snapshot image that pops into our minds of a parent hugging or holding a child or of a child telling his or her parent, "I love you!" In the media, parenthood is often portrayed like a Norman Rockwell painting. When I imagine what I've missed out on by not being a parent, that ideal situation springs up in my imagination. I then have to remind myself that the reality is, of course, a mix of wonderful, awful, boring, and serene.

The adults I've spoken to have shared their intimate and personal experiences in dealing with the idealization of parenting and how this has impacted them. Annie relayed how her grandmother goes on and on about how wonderful it was to have children and how much she enjoyed her role as a mother. Annie shared, "This simply is not the truth. My grandmother suffered from postpartum depression and she had severe bipolar disorder." I've also wondered how adults who don't have kids (myself included) have managed not to fold under the subtle and not so subtle pressures we feel when child rearing is so idealized. People seem to find not having kids to be an unnatural act, while at the same time, procreation is viewed as a miracle.

Marley & Me is a movie that actually presents a fairly balanced view of family living and how having children impacts a marriage. As the story unfolds, the happy couple moves from getting a dog to having three children. The wife in the film, played by Jennifer Aniston, makes a comment at one point about how she never knew it would be so hard. She also laments having lost herself in the process of being a mother. A few Hollywood celebrities are going public with their choice to remain childfree. I was pleased to read recently that actress Cameron Diaz has been speaking out, saying that the planet doesn't need more children, and suggesting that she may never have kids herself. When interviewed by *Cosmopolitan* magazine, she noted, "I think women are afraid to say that they don't want children because they're going to get shunned."[8]

Suzanne, the legal secretary who is childfree by choice, shared that she sometimes finds herself feeling envious of seemingly happy couples with kids, especially in the movies. She explained, "These families typically have a beautiful home, a great car, and nice clothes, and they are often vacationing and everyone is laughing and having a good time. They're frequently seen sharing some intimate moment—teaching the child an important life lesson or some valuable insight." Suzanne expressed sadness, relating, "Missing out on the opportunity to be a mentor or a hero to one's own child seems like a great loss. The imagined intimacy and connection that can only exist between a parent and child makes me wonder if I'm cheating myself. I've seen one of my best friends hug and play with her children and tell them how much she loves them and it makes me feel sad that I won't experience this."

I believe that the idealization of child rearing is related to the natural life force that pushes people to procreate to ensure the survival of the human race. Victoria, a Florida nurse in her fifties who works at Planned Parenthood, sat with me over iced tea in her garden and shared her perceptions on this concept, saying, "When it comes to having children, the conscious part of our being is small compared to the unconscious part. This is a life force that keeps pushing on us all the time. Through the years, although I've felt certain that the right choice for me was to not have children, I've had to keep myself protected. I've learned to find ways to nurture, other than by having kids of my own, and this has helped to keep me armored from the pressure to procreate." Tears began to roll down Victoria's cheeks as she continued to talk. "My mother, may she rest in peace, gave herself up to having children. She didn't seem to have the awareness that she might not be able to handle another child, but she didn't know how to talk with my father about it, or to figure out a way to not keep getting pregnant. By the time her youngest was an adolescent, her mind was so boggled with dealing with too many kids that she resorted to suicide. I think she was drowning emotionally before she decided to drown herself to death that one cold night. She just didn't have the awareness that she could not handle another child and she didn't know how to talk to my father about it or to figure out a way to not keep getting pregnant. In the end, it just wore her down emotionally." After my meeting with Victoria, I felt an enormous sadness for her mother and also for the eight children she left behind, who were unable to enjoy a relationship with their mother in their adult lives. I also had a sense of awe that her mother had readily born and raised so many children, and I wondered about the force within her that seemed to push her to do so.

QUESTIONS TO CONSIDER

Have you experienced babylust or felt the ticking of your biological clock, or have you observed these phenomena in your friends?

What factors may have been behind these phenomena, other than a pure innate drive?

If you've felt a need to nurture, how have you met this?

Have you felt pressure from friends or family to have children?

How have media portrayals of child rearing impacted you?

Do you experience guilt over what your own parents are missing out on as a result of your doubts about having children?

What sacrifices would you have to make if you decided to have children?

What parts of being a parent would you enjoy the most and be the best at?

Have you been accused of being anti-child because you didn't have kids?

What examples of the idealization of child rearing have you been exposed to recently?

What impact, if any, did these idealizations have on you?

Finalizing the Decision

Often, simply going through the experience of information gathering is enough to gain clarity about an important decision. My process involved thinking through all the above factors related to child rearing, looking at the positives and the negatives, and exploring why some situations brought out more emotion in me than others. It was helpful to take some time here to pause and to contemplate it all in depth, rather than pushing it aside as I'd done for so many years. Throughout my life, making important decisions has fallen on opposite ends of the extreme—it's either a long-term process, or it happens almost in the blink of an eye. I've often made decisions regarding relationships very quickly and then moved forward in my commitment with a sense of faith that things will work out. Sometimes they do and other times they don't. In other areas, such as where to move, what kind of job to take, or what kind of dog to adopt, I have spent many months and sometimes years gathering practical data and observing my emotional response over time before taking action.

In a sense, it's been this way with the decision to have or not to have a child. Through the years, from time to time, I'd pull the idea off the shelf and try it on for size. Then, after a day at the most, I'd get busy with a task or turned off to the concept and put it away. I just never quite made a full commitment to it one way or the other, and this led to a lack of closure and periodic doubts. While I always look forward to my quiet evenings after a long day at work, planning adult vacations, and living a fairly simple and uncomplicated life, there have been occasions when I've wondered if I've missed out by not having a child. I'll be out at a park and see a very cute little girl, and think, *Oh, it would be so much fun to spend a couple of hours with her.* The children who bring out this response in me are, of course, well behaved, cute, and very clean. Other times, when I'm walking through a store, a rack of little dresses catches my eye, and I wish for just a moment that I had a daughter of my own to buy one for. I like the idea of being important in a child's life on Mother's Day, of having someone make pancakes for me and honor me in a special way. But these things are simply not reason enough for me to have had a baby. The decision-making process I've experienced is classic—as with anything in life, I've found pros and cons, losses and gains. Our job is to examine all of these factors and to then come to a final answer about what's right for us in the given situation. It's helpful to increase our understanding about what pushes our emotional buttons and to realize that occasional twinges of doubt are normal. It's not unusual to have ambivalence around such huge decisions in life and to even have regrets from time to time about the choices we have made—the problem is when we become stuck in the "what ifs" rather than embracing reality and looking for the positives in our individual circumstances.

Have you taken time to seriously contemplate what it means to be childfree? If not, would it be helpful to do so at this point in your life?

What steps might you take to get started with this process?

The Effects of Doing It All

Once I had gone through the steps above, it was important to bolster my decision with ongoing reminders that life is about choices, and that we simply cannot take all paths. If I'd chosen to become a parent, I would have had less energy to put into my psychology practice and I probably would not have traveled extensively. It's likely that I wouldn't be writing a book. Because getting married and having kids was the most common route to take, many of us who were ambivalent put off making a conscious decision about these huge life choices. This later resulted in second-guessing or regret, even though not having kids has led to other opportunities.

A more recent shift appears to be happening, in that more young people are actually considering whether or not having kids is right for them. These days, among well-educated couples most pregnancies are planned, and the childfree adults I met with shared that family planning is common among their friends. Renee, the university librarian in her early sixties, stated, "In my own group of educated professional people, the decision to have children is taken extremely seriously. Often children are seen as a detriment to career advancement, and the decision to have kids for a woman in a high-pressure career is made with much agonizing, knowing that the gratification of parenting will likely come at some sacrifice to her career." On the other hand, as women, we still are told we can have it all—we can have a successful and fulfilling career and also be a good parent. This can result in a great deal of unhappiness, as many of these mothers rush from the office to pick children up from day care, then work into the night on household and child-rearing tasks. They sacrifice sleep and personal time, and they often do not have the energy to enjoy their career or their role as parent.

The need to carefully contemplate the decision of whether or not to have kids has become more critical as women have moved into more male-dominated positions in the workplace. These jobs cannot be left for a few years and returned to without missing a beat. Women in particular need to carefully assess what they want for themselves and to accept the inherent losses in these decisions. According to *The Observer,* a fifth of women born after 1975 are predicted to remain childfree. Many of these women, if childfree by choice, are unwilling to make the sacrifice to their careers that raising children would take. So, for those who are clear that they want to have children and for those who know they don't, decision making takes place. On the other hand, for those who are ambivalent, chance factors dominate. It's worthwhile to take time to go through a formal decision-making process that may lead to closure and sense of peace with your choice.

QUESTIONS TO CONSIDER

What sacrifices have you not had to make due to not having children?

What are your thoughts on the belief that we can "do it all"?

CHAPTER 3

CHILDFREE PERSONALITIES

"My mom tells me that when I was two, the doctor's records said I was very independent. I've never felt an overwhelming need to have someone around."

—Tracy, age forty-seven

Childfree adults come in many sizes, shapes, and backgrounds—we have no single personality type. Most intentionally childfree adults report that they've always felt they were unique, while many who stumbled into a childfree life by happenstance say that, aside from not being parents, they feel no different from their friends who have kids. One factor that distinguishes childfree adults from their peers with kids is the ability to choose their daily life paths with limited consideration for others—something that is not feasible for most parents. This freedom for the childfree, or lack thereof for parents, has a significant impact on personality development over time. Some people believe that the childfree are somehow flawed, and childfree adults, especially women, are often viewed as cold, selfish, and unwilling to nurture.

Intentionally Childfree Adults

Some childfree adults say they've always known they didn't want to have kids; these men and women have personality qualities that set them apart from the childfree who might have been parents under different life circumstances. A study conducted by professor Christine Brooks examined the personality traits of women she described as *early articulators*: those who have known from an early age that they didn't want to have children.[9] Dr. Brooks conducted in-depth interviews with a number of early articulators and found that they tended to have some very similar characteristics. Most of them prized their autonomy, their ability to maintain control over their environment, and their economic security. These values were viewed as expressions of freedom. These women also strived to contribute to society in some way. They reported both having difficulty relating to women who were mothers and experiencing a loss of friendships when their friends had kids. Some described feeling like outsiders, different from others and judged by women who choose to mother. The majority of women interviewed reported no regret around their decision to not have kids and a high level of satisfaction with their lives. In essence, they prized their freedom and independence, as well as their ability to control their lives.

> **Intentionally childfree adults tend to prize their autonomy, their ability to maintain control over their environment, and their economic security.**

Dr. Brooks's research findings certainly matched up with the stories of the intentionally childfree I interviewed. For example, when I met with Annie, the thirty-three-year-old vocational counselor, she shared, "There's a financial aspect to having kids, and for me it was important to have security and stability. It's a big value to be independent. I notice how a lot of parents these days make their kids the center of their lives and want to be friends with them, too. Because of this, the children don't necessarily want to be independent. I guess my father didn't raise me that way. I was always really excited about being on my own. I remember going out to dinner with my father as a child and seeing women out with their girlfriends all dressed up and buying their own dinner. I wanted to do that myself."

Nicole, the FBI agent, also talked about her strong need for autonomy and independence. She explained, "I'll always look out for myself first and never have to worry that someone else is relying solely on me for survival. Plus, in my line of work there's always the possibility that I could leave for work one day and never come home. I would never put a child through that." You may recall from chapter 1 that both Annie and Nicole were oldest children who were often put in the role of parenting of their younger sisters. The expectation to take on so much responsibility may have played a significant role in their decision to not have kids themselves. I can imagine them as young teenagers, vowing that once they had control over their lives, no one would trap them again.

> "There's a financial aspect to having kids, and for me it was important to have security and stability. It's a big value to be independent."

This need for control and autonomy was also described by childfree by choice adults who were not placed in a parenting role with younger siblings. Suzanne, the legal secretary, shared, "I've always felt different from my peers, even as a child, so it's no surprise that I'm not doing what others are doing. I'm fairly selfish, and I love to move around and to try different things. Plus, I don't have much patience, and I wouldn't want to set myself up for feeling the frustration I think I'd have with children. My friends who are parents seem to have stronger social connections than me—they do things more frequently with their families and friends. I value my freedom and independence, and I don't envy their lives. John and I have lived in Washington State for five years now and before this, we'd only ever lived three years in any given place before moving on. I've moved around so much that I've experienced the impermanence of things. I arrive in a place, and even if I love it, I tell myself that I won't be there forever. Nothing is permanent. I think John is tired of moving around and would like to stay in one place, but I have a stronger will. I thrive on change, new environments, and new activities. When I have to do the same thing over and over again, I feel like I'm going to die."

Diane, the accountant in her early forties, also talked about her need to have control over her life. She shared, "I do believe that Patrick and I are inherently different from adults who have chosen to have kids. We're quite outspoken and in some ways selfish. We aren't afraid of conflict or disagreement. I once overheard someone say that people who didn't have children were missing a sensitivity chip. I'm sure that's not true for everyone, but I actually do believe it to be true of us. We are very compassionate about animals, but have far less tolerance for other humans. My understanding is that when you have children you are forced to become selfless, and we have never had that experience. Our weeknights and weekends belong to us—so we mostly do whatever comes to mind."

"I once overheard someone say that people who didn't have children were missing a sensitivity chip. I'm sure that's not true for everyone, but I actually do believe it to be true of us."

Another common theme among the adults I heard from was their strong desire to continue to develop and grow and not to lose their personal sense of self. Annie's husband Roger shared, "On Mondays I talk to people at work about how their weekends went. I want to have something interesting about my life to share that represents what I do and what I think about. When people say that they went to their child's soccer game, I find myself wanting to interrupt and ask them about *their* weekend, not their child's weekend. I have a strong emotional reaction when a parent's entire weekend is about their child. I don't hold it against them, but I somehow feel sad for them. I wonder if, at a certain point, perhaps twenty-five years down the road, there's going to be anything going on in their lives." Annie interjected her thoughts on the matter, adding, "We watch *What Not to Wear*, and most of the participants are mothers who have lost everything about themselves in the process of being moms."

Roger and Annie are vibrant, attractive, and physically strong and healthy. When they arrived at my office they shared that Annie had walked and Roger had brought their car. I observed their obvious independence as a couple, each engaging in activities of their own, but the emotional bond between them was apparent through their close eye contact and the way they casually completed thoughts for one another at times during the interview. There were other times, however, when they disagreed, and they were able to allow this, too. Nicole also described her mission of personal growth. "I try to make sure I'm always moving forward, never letting my life become stale. I tend to have a ready supply of educational, health, work, travel, and relationship goals."

"My coworkers with children use the kids as an excuse to not work certain shifts, or to take time off from work. Can you imagine if I took the day off because my dog was sick or I needed to take him to the vet?"

Another strong theme Nicole addressed was the importance of taking personal responsibility for herself, and she observed that parents sometimes use having kids as an excuse for not doing so. She explained, "I've thought from time to time that many people have kids so that they don't have to take further steps to improve themselves. Once the kids arrive, everything in their own lives is put on hold and their entire focus is on their children. I don't have that. If I decide not to continue to improve myself I can never use the excuse that my kids come first. So many parents I know say they want things for themselves but follow it up by saying they may do these things when the kids get older. That's bullshit. I also notice that many of my friends with children become consumed in the kids' activities and then no longer feel pressured to succeed, having transferred that pressure." Nicole complained about how her colleagues used this to their advantage, "My coworkers with children use the kids as an excuse to not work certain shifts, or to take time off from work. Can you imagine if I took the day off because my dog was sick or I needed to take him to the vet?"

In some social circles, it might actually be considered the norm to stay home from work to care for a sick pet, but in many family-focused communities, including the city where I live, this is scoffed at. I recently had a childfree patient call to cancel her appointment because she needed to stay home to care for her ill cat. As a pet owner who views my dog as my child, I felt that this was a perfectly legitimate reason for canceling her appointment, but one of my secretaries, who is a mother, had a haughty reaction, saying, "Can you believe she's canceling her appointment because her cat is sick?"

> "I think I am different. I'm not as tolerant as others, and I'm not afraid to tell people how I feel about things."

Arno, the retired respiratory therapist, also talked about feeling frustrated with parents getting special treatment and his strong belief that people should take personal responsibility. When I met with him over coffee, I immediately noted from his outward appearance that he was different—neatly dressed in jeans and a button-down shirt, he wore his long hair pulled back in a ponytail. I listened with interest as he shared his story. "I think I am different. I'm not as tolerant as others, and I'm not afraid to tell people how I feel about things. For example, if I noticed someone doing something that seemed out of line, I wouldn't think twice about getting up and saying something to them about their behavior. I'm willing to take responsibility for myself, and I think that others should do the same, even parents. I can't believe it when I see special parking spaces marked for parents with young children. What about making accommodations for folks who haven't intentionally caused the struggles they're asking to be compensated for?"

Both Nicole and Arno expressed some resentment towards parents, seeming to take on an attitude of, "They made their bed and should now lie in it!" It's debatable exactly how much special treatment and compensation ought to be given to someone simply because he or she is a parent. Perhaps in the past, when there was justification for bringing more people into the world, this might have made sense, but these days, when we actually need to decrease the world population, it seems logical for parents to take full responsibility for their decisions.

While reflecting on the words of these adults who are childfree by choice, I was reminded of the concept of *locus of control*. This is a psychological term that describes whether or not a person feels in control over her destiny. An individual with an *internal locus of control* believes that she is in charge of the direction of her life. On the other hand, a person with an *external locus of control* views life as something that simply happens; she's taken on a ride and has little say over where she will end up.

> **An individual with an internal locus of control believes that she is in charge of the direction of her life. On the other hand, a person with an external locus of control views life as something that simply happens; she's taken on a ride and has little say over where she will end up.**

When I asked Suzanne about her sense of this in herself, she responded, "I try to control what I can, because life is chaotic and whatever I can control, I do. I try to live consciously and I spend too much time thinking about my life and what life means. I do well with living in the moment, but I don't want to be on remote control—a part of this is about making conscious decisions and examining my life and deciding what direction I want to go in. I feel that my life has been an example of passion, intent, and purpose. I tell friends and family what my goals are, and then I tend to make them happen. I love to be spontaneous about inconsequential decisions but not about the big things, like having a baby."

The statistic that over half the women in the United States become pregnant without planning to do so provides a great example of allowing your life to unfold as it may. Jill, the forty-three-year-old network engineer, shared a story along these lines. "I used to work with Lucy, a young woman in her early twenties. Lucy had recently gotten married and she told me that she was going to stop using contraception. I said, 'So, you're planning to get pregnant?' Lucy said, 'No. I'm open to it but not planning it.' A few days later I happened to be at a gathering with some of my women friends, and I asked them if they thought this young woman should plan her pregnancy or just allow it to happen. The answers were across the board. Some said that if you didn't plan it you'd just die, because it was so hard. Others said that being a parent was the best thing that had ever happened to them, and that their pregnancy had been a complete surprise." Jill's social circle of well-educated women who acknowledged that many of their pregnancies were not planned flies in the face of the idea that this only happens to immature teens. I personally believe that, although they are reticent to admit it, many otherwise responsible people become pregnant by accident, simply because they did not make *not* getting pregnant a top priority. The early articulators I met with, and those interviewed by Christine Brooks, had prioritized that an unplanned pregnancy did not happen for them. In general they seemed to be more goal focused, and, in a sense, more controlling than the average person. A part of their decision not to have kids included the fact that children are unpredictable, and parents must forego their sense of needing to be in control all the time.

QUESTIONS TO CONSIDER

Do childfree adults have a greater need for independence and control than parents?

Is there a correlation between internal versus external locus of control and choosing to be childfree?

What is your locus of control? Are you driving or sitting in the passenger's seat of the car of life?

The Impact of Being Childfree on Personality Development over Time

It's only logical that a person who doesn't have kids would wind up being more independent than one who becomes a parent, simply given the enormous amount of time and emotional energy children take. My twenties, thirties, and forties—the years when, had I been a parent, my children would likely have arrived and been raised—have been hugely formative for me. I've tended to want to do things my own way since high school, and over time this desire and the resultant independent lifestyle became polished and more distinctive. As a young adult, I began to make a series of choices that moved me further and further away from the mainstream, such as moving away from the South, traveling the world on my own, and getting a PhD. As I took each of these steps, my sense of being different from others grew, and so too did my need for constant change, growth, and control over my life. My self-perception as a psychologist, a romantic partner, and an adventure-seeker who thrives on goals also became clearer over time, as did my priority of living my daily life in such a way that my actions match the image I have of myself. My personal life is fairly self-focused, with no one else to consider other than Chris and Bella. Even still, it's difficult for me to put my own desires first, above what I think would make Chris and Bella happy. So I can only imagine that, as a parent, my primary focus would be on my child. I'd be so busy taking care of the tasks involved in this role that there might not be much left for me.

Much has been written about how motherhood changes people, and I've witnessed this with my own group of friends. When I connected to Facebook, I began to find out what was happening with all kinds of people from my past who I hadn't heard from for many years. Most of them had photographs of their children on their pages, and their daily updates were heavily focused on what they'd done with their kids the day before. Some of them shared quite personal information about their children, including how many universities they'd been accepted to, and I couldn't help but wonder how the children felt about this. In Peggy Orenstein's *Waiting for Daisy*, she writes about her experience prior to her daughter's birth, when most of her girlfriends are having children. Nearly all of them have dropped out of the workforce and seem obsessed with their children's daily lives. Peggy notes that they seem to her, at times, to be like something out of *Invasion of the Body Snatchers*! Some are content, but most seem trapped, worrying about what they will do once the children are older. They appear to be hesitant to assert their own needs, as doing so might disrupt their husbands' careers.

Motherhood does cause some women to lose their ambition. My former colleague Janelle was an adamant feminist, but when she became pregnant she decided to take an extended leave from her career to be a stay at home mom. This resulted in her being financially dependent on her husband, and when she returned to work several years later, she complained about not being promoted at the same pace as those of us who had remained on the job all along. Janelle also showed through her actions that work was not a top priority; she often left work early to attend children's events or stayed home with sick children.

Watching your friends change once a baby arrives can be disturbing. Rachel Cooke wrote a February 2009 article for *The Guardian* in which she describes the sense of horror and fear she feels when she encounters "dummy mummies,"[10] or mothers who go on and on about the most trivial events in their children's lives and are excessively focused on strollers, breastfeeding, and bedtime routines.

On a similar note, Suzanne shared, "I can't rely on my children's lives to identify me. My life is my own and ultimately it's up to me to generate my own happiness. There are times when I'm in the midst of friends who have kids and I feel alienated, but for the most part I'm proud to tell people about the various things I do or have done in order to quickly identify myself rather than just saying, 'I have two kids, ages blah and blah, who are into such and such . . .' I truly enjoy having the freedom in my life to work on personal growth, and I usually like to talk about these things with others. At times, though, I think it would be nice not to have to put such an effort into my own life and instead totally focus on someone else's life, like my child's. Having a kid would give me a legitimate excuse to take a break from my own personal growth."

> "I can't rely on my children's lives to identify me. My life is my own and ultimately it's up to me to generate my own happiness."

Mark, the Seattle engineer, also noted that he's observed the way parents wrap their lives around their children's, explaining, "I have a coworker, Josh, who has three boys, nine, seven, and five. He's very focused at work and also at home, but man, there is little else. Another guy has a six-year-old and twin two-year-old monsters. They have their own family web page. These guys seem almost drugged by fatherhood, which is great for them—they seem enthralled and totally consumed by it. I can't imagine myself in that position. I wonder what will happen to them once the children are grown."

Others talked about how not having kids has impacted their self-perception. Diane, the accountant, shared, "I think both Patrick and I are many things—we're committed, honest, hard working, animal lovers, and motorcycle enthusiasts. Being childfree hasn't impacted our identity—it has simply shifted it in a different direction because we have time to devote to our passions that we wouldn't have if we were parents."

How have you changed during the years that might otherwise have been spent raising children?

Have you had more or less change compared with your friends who are parents?

What are the primary differences between you and your friends who are parents?

Having Fun and the Fear of Losing Youthfulness

I recently had a dream in which Chris and I were sitting at a table in a café. The waitress brought over our food, placed my plate in front of me, and said, "Here you are, Granny." In the dream, I was appalled. First, I looked at Chris and then said to the woman, "I'm not a grandmother!"—as if I'd been accused of having some kind of disease. The dream was a perfect reflection of my resolve not to turn into the stereotypical middle-aged woman who has allowed herself to grow plump, wear dowdy clothing, and lost all interest in sex and romance. This is, of course, not the case for all grandmothers, but the idea that it might happen to me clashes with my aspiration of being more like Sophia Loren, who is sexy in her older years.

Some of the adults I met with also talked about their yearning to remain youthful. Mark, the engineer, stated, "If I had it to do over, I wouldn't want to relive the exact same life. I know I'd start playing golf as a boy instead of waiting until I was forty-seven, that's for sure. One of the things Sarah and I love about not having kids is having a double income and the freedom to do what we want with our time and our money. I sure wouldn't give that up."

Some would read Mark's words and judge him as selfish and immature, and indeed, childfree adults are sometimes described as fun people who never quite grew up. Trish, a sixty-five-year-old psychotherapist, told me about her mother's only sister, Aunt Melba, who never had children. "I watched how Aunt Melba didn't have kids and how she had the time to be very active in my life. She was always the fun aunt, but she was also very self-focused and not at all serious about important things in life."

Others talked about their need to both enjoy life and to do something meaningful. Carrie the medical biller shared, "At this point in my life, I'm just having fun, but I'd like to do something other than just work forty hours a week. I don't know what it is. I'm not sure what my mission in life is. I'm still exploring and thinking about doing things. I'd like to volunteer, but I just don't have the time or the energy to do that yet. I'm rolling through my life having fun, and before you know it I'll be eighty years old."

Because we, the childfree, don't have the identity of being a parent, it's easier for us not to shift into that mature, adult persona that seems to overtake people once they have a child. My observation is that childfree adults are more playful and less serious than our peers who have children. The most obvious reason for this is simply the lack of responsibility for another being who is vulnerable and totally dependent. This responsibility can certainly bring joy, but it is also undeniably a burden, and once a child is born, parents often never stop having parental concerns, even once that child is living his or her own life as an adult.

QUESTIONS TO CONSIDER

Are you more concerned about remaining youthful than your friends who have children?

Do you have concerns about not having anyone dependent on you?

Are Childfree Adults Cold and Selfish?

I suppose it's not unusual for parents who are crazy about their kids, and for adults who are really into children in general, to view with suspicion those who have chosen a childfree life. Unfortunately, this perception seems to be growing, as is the divide between the childfree and parents. Parents are often left awestruck when adults say out loud that their childfree status is actually by choice, and that they never experienced the babylust they observe in others. I was recently at a party where I found myself in the kitchen chatting about my interviews for this book with a woman in her fifties whom I'd never met before. She was quite eager to tell me about her recent experience with an old friend, saying, "I recently had the most bizarre experience! My best friend is a woman in her fifties who never had children. She was here a few weeks ago for a visit, and I brought her over to meet my three-week-old grandson. I asked her to hold the baby, and she did so for just a minute before handing the child back over to me. When I asked again if she wanted to hold the baby, she insisted that she really didn't want to and that she wasn't interested in doing so. I felt confused and astounded. I simply can't understand why she wouldn't have any interest in holding my grandson."

Many would jump to the conclusion that because a woman isn't interested in babies, she is inherently cold, not nurturing, and unfeminine—all qualities that childfree women would argue do not depend solely on motherhood. In the words of actress and comedian Janeane Garofalo, "I thought in the past that I wanted to have children, but now I realize that I don't. People think that you are a nasty, selfish person if you don't want to have children."

Although I haven't been told I'm nasty, I've had friends tell me that I'm the hardest working woman they know, and that I'm both competitive and ambitious. These are not especially flattering descriptions for a woman, at least not for a Southern Belle like myself, but I suppose I must appear this way to an outsider looking in. I truly think that a huge part of what makes me who I am is my energy level, which I inherited from my mother. At seventy-six years old, she is up at 5:30 each morning to do chores around her farm or to read and have quiet time for herself. She tends to be on the go all day long and to get a huge amount done. I'm much the same way, getting up early even on weekends and preferring to be productive and busy rather than lounging around. At work, I'm focused and able to push through efficiently. I don't really think these character traits are related to not having kids. Despite my industriousness, I see myself as quite nurturing, both at work and at home. As a therapist, I provide empathy and support to patients every day, and at home I am nurturing to Bella and Chris and to our friends, who I love to entertain.

Other childfree women have similar views of themselves. Jill, the network engineer, shared, "I often feel that I'm different from other women, but it's not necessarily something that they notice. I believe that if any of my friends who didn't know that I had intentionally chosen to not be a parent were asked if I had the characteristics of a natural mother, they would say that I would be a great mom, because I have a lot of nurturing qualities. Most people have no idea that I'm not particularly interested in being nurturing with children. I love the company of adults and that's where I spend most of my time. I have plenty of friends who have kids, but I choose not to spend much time with them. I'm very much a caretaker of my partner, Susan, and my friends. I've often thought that if I'd had kids I would have given so much that I would have shrunk and shrunk and ultimately disappeared. I suppose it's because my parents modeled a lot of giving, so the bar was set high.

This, combined with my tendency to over-function, would have been problematic."

Jill also commented on the suggestion by some that childfree adults are selfish. She noted, "I don't think people with kids realize how my life is. I just don't know how they juggle it all. Something has got to give, and I'm unwilling to give up career, friends, my relationship with Susan, or time for myself. I read the book *The Feminine Mistake* [Voice/Hyperion, 2007], by Leslie Bennetts, who wrote about the decision to leave the workforce and to raise children. She lays out statistics in her book on the likelihood of it all working out okay. It's like we fuss over all these little decisions and don't fuss over the big ones. I feel absolutely no guilt about not being as busy as my friends who are parents—luckily, I shed that Midwestern mentality long ago." Other women I spoke with echoed Jill's sentiments. Diane, the accountant, shared, "Without a doubt, I have never felt guilty about having more free time than my friends with children. I love my free time. I love sleeping in or snuggling in bed with a good book or a movie on a rainy day."

"Without a doubt, I have never felt guilty about having more free time than my friends with children. I love my free time."

Being nurturing and feminine is not synonymous with having children. Many of the women I interviewed describe themselves as giving and warm with their friends and family, but this does not necessarily mean they have a desire to use these qualities with children. This is yet another example of the societal expectation that women are linked with children. When there are no children in the picture, we are not viewed in the same way, even though we may be extremely nurturing and giving with our pets, our friends, our family, and in our professional lives. When a woman says she doesn't have kids, some people make instant assumptions about her. Dr. Caroline Gatrell conducted research on women in employment and found that some bosses consider those who choose not to have kids to be cold and odd, and refuse to promote them, viewing their lack of maternal instinct as a lack of "essential humanity."[11]

It may be that adults who don't have children are actually more compassionate and sensitive than many parents. A great example of this is Carrie, who shared, "Steven says that I would have died a thousand deaths if I'd had kids because I would have felt every pain with them. My mom never put pressure on me to have children, and I don't think she enjoyed raising us. I think she felt too much for us, and she felt too much pressure, and she believes that I would have felt my children's pain the way she did."

QUESTIONS TO CONSIDER

Have you been accused of being selfish because you don't have children?

How do you nurture others in your life?

Feeling Different

Some people march to the beat of a different drum. Since high school, if not earlier, I have felt that I was inherently different from my peers. Many of the childfree adults I interviewed for this book reported that they also feel different from others—plus, they often feel like outsiders.

Jackie the paralegal, took a different stance, insisting that she is not different from her peers with kids. She explained, "When I get together with my friends who have children, and the kids aren't there, they're back to their old selves. One difference between us, though, is that I don't think I could spend the rest of my life with one man in my home with little children running around the house—that thought is not pleasant. I like my single life." Jackie did, however, tell me that she feels left out at times when she is with a group of mothers. She recalled, "Because I've always lived next door to my sister and helped her out quite a bit in raising her daughter, I've gone with them to many social gatherings through the years. I can't tell you how often I've felt ignored by the mothers there, almost like they felt that I didn't have the right to be there or that I was invisible. I can't even put into words how this made me feel; it was really awful. I wonder, in retrospect, if these mothers felt that I was criticizing or judging them. I suppose I'll never know."

Jackie's words bring to light some concerning speculations. I truly feel that the divide between parents and the childfree, particularly for women, is growing, because we are so misunderstood and even at times mistrusted by mothers. We may find ourselves, from time to time, in a position of having to put forth extra effort not to be perceived as critical and cold. The key is being able to talk openly about the life choice to not have kids and the hope of reaching a point in our culture in which this is embraced as a positive choice that results in energy available for other nurturing venues.

QUESTIONS TO CONSIDER

Have you felt shunned when in a group of mothers?

What steps have you taken, if any, to demonstrate your acceptance of children?

CHAPTER 4
CHILDFREE DAYS

"I have so many friends who live in small houses in south London with all these babies underfoot and it's just not attractive. I'm selfish and I can't bear mess and ugliness and those things come hand-in-hand with children."

—Hugh Grant, actor

Life without children is dramatically different from family living. First of all, there's the abundance of free time. Couples without kids have more opportunity to be together without the distractions of caring for children. The way childfree adults experience their weekends and holidays is also quite different.

Weeknight Bliss

When you don't have children, every day can feel like a Friday, with a hard day at the office followed by a relaxing, self-indulgent, and rejuvenating evening. I wonder if a true Friday ever comes for parents, always faced with hungry mouths to feed, laundry, and an overwhelming number of other tasks to do. A person without kids can generally defer household tasks to the next day; after all, no one else is impacted.

As a childfree adult, I've come to relish my non-scheduled workday evenings. Chris and I usually work until 6:30 and then we come home and go for a run or work on our individual projects. Most evenings I enjoy taking half an hour to myself with a glass of wine and a bowl of nuts while I read the latest issue of *Bon Appétit*. If I have energy, I might take a few minutes to balance the checkbook or to pay a few bills. I begin making dinner around 7:30, mulling over what I'd like to prepare. I like to make healthy, simple meals such as broiled salmon with brown rice and salad. My time in the kitchen is quiet and creative. While I cook, Chris does his own thing, and we reconvene once dinner is ready.

Talk to most childfree adults and you'll find that they relish their leisure time and flexibility in their daily schedules. For most of us, ordinary weekdays are a time of self-focus and indulgence. Nobody I spoke to talked about feeling lonely or bored—even those childfree adults who are single and living alone.

Jackie, the single paralegal, told me about a typical workday evening. "I get off work at 5 pm and then go home and have whatever I want for dinner; I really don't put much focus on making a well-balanced meal." She laughed, admitting, "I went through a phase when I had ice cream for dinner every night. I love living alone and being responsible only for my own chores. I come home to an empty house, and if it's messy, it's my mess, and if it's clean, it's my clean!" As Jackie chuckled, I recalled that when we'd discussed where we should meet for our interview, she'd stated clearly that her condo was not an option because it was too cluttered for her to have guests. "Some nights after dinner, I exercise, and on other evenings, I meet up with a girlfriend, and we go out to Starbucks. Then I watch television or spend some time organizing. I really just spend my evenings doing whatever I want to do."

> "My weeknights are taken with me-centered activities, such as volunteer work or creative pursuits—things that my friends with kids only get to do on a limited basis."

Other childfree adults use their evening time to earn extra money. Denise, the office manager who's also single, noted, "I work until around 5 pm, and I like to exercise right after work. I get home at around 6 pm and then I get going with my second job, transcription, typing until 8:30. Because it's just me, I have the energy and time to put in a couple of hours of work in the evening, and I like having the extra money. My friends who have children say I work too hard, but to me, it seems like I have plenty of time for a second job and fun too!" She added, "I splurge on having a housekeeper who comes in every week for a couple of hours, so I have very little housework to do for myself each week. I have dinner late, at 8:30, and then do something fun and relaxing until bedtime at 11 pm. I enjoy doing a creative project, such as scrapbooking, collaging, card making, knitting, or needlework. I also sell baby hats on the side. If I'm not being creative, I like to read, watch television, and play with my cat. If I had children to care for, I might have had to give up my creative endeavors or limit them."

Denise added that over the years she's observed just how different her evenings are from those of her girlfriends with children. "My weeknights are taken with me-centered activities, such as volunteer work or creative pursuits—things that my friends with kids only get to do on a limited basis."

Writer Nancy Rome describes just how different daily life is for childfree adults in her 2006 article for the *Washington Post*, in which she writes, "Those of us who are not mothers do not fit into any of society's convenient boxes: We're not slaves to carpools or homework. At the same time, we are not necessarily obsessed about our careers or even ourselves; nor are we anti-family. Our days are simply lived according to a different rhythm: Children don't tug at my clothes and beg for attention; I don't leave my cell phone on during films or dinner parties in case the babysitter needs me; I travel; I read books—lots of them—as well as the newspaper."[12]

Jackie and Denise both seem to be quite content in their lives, despite not having children and not having partners. What personality traits protect them from feeling bored or lonely?

How do your evenings compare to those of your friends who have children?

Date Night Every Night

The childfree couples I talked to tend to have evenings rich with together-time. Their stories are quite different from those I hear in my office from couples with children, who try to schedule a date night every week or two. Many childfree couples have date night almost every night. Suzanne, the legal secretary who is married to John, shared, "We value not having to divide our evening time with other people or activities. Our time together is absolutely our own. After work, we create and share a meal together, talk about the day, watch a movie, or play a game. Sometimes John reads while I work on an art project."

For Mark and Sarah, the professional couple in their fifties, most evenings are quiet by design. "We enjoy being in our home with each other. We always eat a respectable dinner, and then we read together in our little reading room. It's a real treat to go to bed early to snuggle or enjoy leisurely lovemaking."

A common complaint from couples with children is about the infrequency of sex, either due to fatigue or to difficulty finding uninterrupted time. In a survey of 5,000 women in 2003, more than 54 percent reported a loss of sexual appetite for up to six months after their children were born.[13]

Our close friends, Marie and Sam, have established a fun

evening routine; Marie enjoys preparing a gourmet candlelit dinner for the two of them every night of the week, and they spend a couple of hours each evening at the table relishing the feast she has created.

Chris and I also have a nice arrangement of sharing meals; he makes breakfast for the two of us every morning while I savor my coffee and newspaper, and I prepare our dinner each evening. It's a treat to live with someone who appreciates my cooking and eats with gusto. Over dinner we like to chat about our day, gossip a bit, flirt, or talk about what we're looking forward to doing over

"I have a lot of control over how I spend my time."

the weekend. It's fun to occasionally allow Bella to jump up into my lap or to sneak her a bite from my plate. After dinner, we enjoy going for a stroll with Bella around the neighborhood, even if it's raining. One of my favorite times of the day is crawling into bed with a good book or my laptop and winding down for a half an hour before falling asleep.

Jill, the network engineer who lives with her partner, Susan, described the pace of her evenings. "My evenings are incredibly leisurely. This becomes even more apparent to me each day at lunch when I hear my colleagues with kids talk about what they did the night before. They will have gone to a soccer game or helped a child with a school project, while I'll have gone for a walk after work, read a book, taken a bath, or watched a movie. Susan and I enjoy a really quiet home and our lives follow a simple routine. My days involve getting up and going to work, working hard, and doing my evening thing and going to bed. I have a lot of control over how I spend my time."

Carrie, the married medical biller, shared that she always looks forward to evenings at home. "It's my favorite time of the day. I love to cook, and I love being at home at night with my husband Steven. We have a nice dinner every night. He's on his laptop computer in the kitchen while I cook and so we're together. We like to eat dinner late. I don't like to just throw a Lean Cuisine on the table. I grow my own herbs, and it's fun to make a big pasta dish with chicken or fish and a nice salad. Spending time slicing and dicing everything by hand is my way of unwinding after a busy day at work. I like to have a glass of wine and take my time. After dinner, we go to our bedroom to watch TV, because it's the coziest room in our home. I go to bed at 10 pm, because I'm pretty beat during the week."

Laurie the engineer told me about her evenings, saying that she and her husband Craig have dinner together at home most nights. Laurie works a 4/10 schedule and because Craig is self-employed, he's able to set his own work schedule so that they can maximize their time together. She shared, "I lift weights some nights after work and one evening a week I play on a soccer team."

As I interviewed couples, I wondered if any of them were in marital therapy. Based on the reported quantity and quality of their time together, I doubted it. In my work with couples who are struggling in their relationships, a common homework assignment is simply to get them to commit to spending more time together. Friendships cannot grow without that commitment. Couples with children usually put the kids first; they sometimes work opposite schedules in order to keep the children out of day care, resulting in a sacrifice of time together. The couples who participated in my project spend most evenings at home, and then enjoy quiet meals together; this is a logical formula for intimacy.

QUESTIONS TO CONSIDER

Do your ordinary evenings feel like date nights?

How do your weeknights compare with those of your friends who have children?

Weekends Are for Fun!

It's become a pattern for Chris and me to be at home most evenings during the week and to do the bulk of our socializing on the weekends. We enjoy going out to a nice restaurant for light dinner and a drink at the bar on Friday nights. We sometimes invite a friend or two to join us, but most often we relish being alone. After dinner, we often rent a movie. Chris and I both have trouble sleeping in on Saturday, because we're excited about having the entire day to do whatever we please. For me, that's usually working on my book project and then going out grocery shopping or doing some yard work. On Saturday evenings, we like to go out to a movie or invite friends over for dinner, especially if we've both been busy with projects all day.

Carrie told me about the Friday night ritual of going out with best friends that she and Steven have established. Afterward, they spend most of the weekend alone together. Carrie noted, "Steven is really fun, and we're each other's favorite person to spend time with. We're always on the go on the weekend and I really believe that if we'd had children, we would be stuck at home. My relationship with Steven has been all about fun!"

Childfree adults aren't at the soccer field on Saturday mornings, unless they choose to be there. Denise shared that she's always gotten together with friends who have kids, going to soccer games or participating in other family activities, and she's found pleasure in sharing in those experiences. Of course if it's raining, she can opt out! She added that she spends her weekends running errands, doing social things with friends and family, and working at her typing job. I asked her if she felt any guilt about having more free time than her friends with children. "Heck no!" she replied. "My free time is full with things I choose to fill it with, and sometimes I wish had more of it."

Renee, the librarian from Nashville, shared, "Now that my friends with kids are empty-nesters, and they have their lives back, my weekends have once again become ridiculously busy, filled with all kinds of fun activities." Her comment caused me to think about the times when I've found myself looking ahead to the day when my friends' children are grown, so that they will once again be free to come out and play with me.

On weekends, childfree couples tend to share house cleaning and chores, but there's also time for fun. Mark and Sarah love to walk, ski, bike, and golf together, and they have a ritual of going out to breakfast every Friday and Saturday morning. Mark told me, "We're comfortable going our own way and being alone, but mostly we're joined at the hip and we love it. Although we have a lot of interaction with Sarah's family, including her sisters and nieces and nephews, we treasure our time with each other most of all."

"I feel like my house is a place where, for children, fun goes to die, because when friends come over with their kids, they're constantly saying, 'no.' It's not a very child-friendly place."

Laurie shared, "Typical weekend activities for Craig and me are motorcycle riding, camping, hiking, going to car shows, working around the house, and visiting with friends or family. Sometimes we do things together; sometimes we go our own way. Very rarely do we do things with people who have kids, and outings with children aren't repeated if we don't like the kids."

Diane and her partner Patrick recently enjoyed going to San Juan Island for the day on their motorcycles. Diane shared, "We spent the day riding around the island, had a great lunch, ate ice cream at the pier and wandered around the shops downtown. We could have made the trip with children, but not with the motorcycles, and I'm guessing the focus would have been centered on entertaining the kids rather than ourselves. While having dogs limits us to taking day trips unless we plan ahead, we can really do whatever we want, whenever we want. We love having that freedom!"

Suzanne smiled as she shared, "John and I spend our weekends taking the dog for a hike or running errands. Sometimes we hang out at a coffee shop. We might also visit with friends or work on things we didn't have time to get to during the week, such as finances, chores, and home repairs. Most often we enjoy sleeping in, having leisurely mornings sipping coffee and talking, and evenings drinking wine and just enjoying each other's company."

QUESTIONS TO CONSIDER

What is your favorite way to spend the weekend?

How do your weekends differ from those of your friends and colleagues who are parents?

What's an Ordinary Day?

Many intentionally childfree adults live unique lives, with careers or schedules that are quite different from the 9-to-5 lives that many people lead. "I don't have an ordinary day and I've never had an ordinary day!" exclaimed Arno, the retired respiratory therapist. "I started working night shift many years ago. Even though I haven't worked for several years now, I still go to bed at 4 am and wake up whenever I wake up, sometime in the early afternoon."

FBI agent Nicole shared, "I work a lot! I work weekends, so a typical Tuesday is no different for me than a typical Saturday."

Tracy, the web designer who works at home, said that she gets up and has breakfast and then works for as long as she can, until 2 or 3 in the afternoon. "If the weather is bad, I'll go to the gym, and if it's good I garden or go for a bike ride. I work for six or seven hours straight without a break, even to eat. This works well for me." Tracy admitted that the transition between day and evening is a tough time for her. She's found it helpful to get more involved in the lives of her friends whose children participate in activities that take place around that time. "I make a concerted effort to be involved in my friends' kids' lives. That means a lot to me and to them also. I'm an aunt by choice. For example, I go with one friend to the pool a couple of evenings a week; we sit by the pool and visit while her son swims. Another friend has a son who plays basketball, and I enjoy going to his games. These things get me out of the house and keep me from being too isolated. I spend most of my time, probably 90 percent, alone. On the weekends, I sometimes go to a potluck or out with friends, but after about two hours I'm ready to come home. I'm definitely an introvert." She added, "I have a lot of time to think and I need that time. I'm a solitary person. I work alone and I live alone. When people ask me if I have kids, I say 'no.' They usually don't have much to say about it after that! It's like they feel sorry for me because I live a quiet life alone. They just assume that I'm lonely since I don't have a husband or kids." Tracy laughed as she described her home, saying, "I feel like my house is a place where, for children, fun goes to die, because when friends come over with their kids, they're constantly saying, 'no.' It's not a very child-friendly place."

I wonder how Tracy really feels about how her friends' children don't enjoy visiting her home and if other childfree adults have this same experience. Her comments brought a smile to my face, as our house is definitely not childproof! It's an adult playground of white carpet, floor-to-ceiling glass, and a deck with a thin cable railing that a small child might try to squeeze his body through. In the two years we've lived here, not a single child has come through the front door—not because I don't *like* children, but because Chris and I have surrounded ourselves with friends who either don't have kids or whose kids are grown up. The more time I spend in this calm, quiet space, the more I crave it and the less I like chaos and noise.

Does your life have non-structured elements because you don't have kids?

Is your home a child-friendly place, or is it an adult playground?

Special Days

> *"I think what you've never had you never miss and I've never had a family Christmas . . . it's always been a twosome. I know it's a naughty thing to say but I don't feel deprived. I've been asked in the past and said I'm sure I'll regret it someday but I must confess I haven't. I don't think the world would be a better place if there were lots of little Whickers running about."*
> —Alan Whicker, TV host/documentarian

Childfree adults have mixed feelings about holidays. Suzanne shared, "I went alone to visit my family this year for the holidays. I missed my husband a lot. Over the Christmas break, I typically look for activities where people will be together. In past years, we've gone out to a local pub, where there is a celebration and special dinner. We also like to get together with other people who don't have children. I focus on crafts, baking, cooking, and sending gifts to others, but sometimes it's hard to create the "magic" without having children around. I noticed, however, that when I was with my family this past year, even though there were children around, it wasn't magical. People were tired and cranky and argumentative, and there was a lot of drama. I was sad because I missed my husband and my dog. I've honestly come to feel a little desperate about having some rituals in place for special days like Christmas and birthdays—because our families live in another state, and so we really are isolated. I just try to keep busy and to find places to go to celebrate where others are also celebrating."

Holidays can be an emotional time for a lot of people. It's hard for me to be so far away from my family, and spending time with other people's families just doesn't meet that special need. I've discovered over the last couple of years that it feels great to get out of town, and Chris and I have created our own ritual of going skiing on Christmas Day. This year, as we were driving home from our skiing holiday, I began to think about how my holiday season is so very different because I am not a mother. I loved planning Christmas Eve dinner for a group of adults and it was great to do a minimal amount of shopping for gifts and to not have to go to a single toy store. On Christmas Day we woke up early, went for a nice run, and had some wonderful leftovers for breakfast of lamb chops, scalloped potatoes, and salad. We ate, packed the car and left for a four-day ski trip in Idaho. There were no early morning Santa preparations and we didn't spend the day serving everyone and putting toys together. I realize that for some, these Christmas rituals are delightful, but I was very happy to be heading out of town.

Chris and I had a quiet, relaxing day going just where we wanted to go, and we spent Christmas night in a fancy bar in Spokane eating hamburgers and Caesar salads. I imagine that if we had children, the trip would have been focused on them, where they wanted to go, and what they wanted to do. It certainly would have lacked romance, and I would have felt exhausted from trying to make sure that everyone was happy. I likely would have worried about how much money was being spent on every little thing for the four days that we were away. There would no doubt have been arguing between siblings or defiance towards adults, and I would have spent much of the weekend playing referee. I remember quite clearly the family vacations we took when I was growing up. My memories of those times are filled with moments of joy and angst, and I recall that the focus was always on what would be pleasing to my brother and me, rather than on what my parents might have preferred. Looking back, I realize how much of a sacrifice my parents made, and it makes me both sad and appreciative. Now, when they come to visit, I get a lot of pleasure out of planning our activities and meals around what they will most enjoy.

Denise shared that because she has made an effort to have children in her life in various ways, it's made holiday times special for her. Every year she invites over one of her friends with children and they help decorate her Christmas tree. She's often involved in their holiday festivities as Aunt Denise. "I love purchasing gifts for them," she tells me. "My sister's children, even though we live in different cities, have been a joy for me also. At Christmastime, my family always gets together at Mom's house. My two sisters with children bring their families, and my other childfree sister is there, as well as Mom. We love to play games, go to a movie, cook and eat, and open gifts. It's been fun to watch the kids grow."

For Tracy, Hanukkah is a special time that she spends alone with her elderly parents. "My parents have a condo in town and my brothers both have families. My parents come out here for the holidays. They're eighty-two and I'm not sure what I'll do when they're gone." Diane and Patrick also spend the holidays with family. Diane shared, "Patrick isn't really close to his parents or to his siblings, and because we don't have kids, there's less sense of obligation to get together with them on the holidays. We usually spend Christmas Eve with my parents and then enjoy being at home alone on Christmas Day."

Nicole has a contrary experience, as she is not with family over the holidays. She shared, "I usually volunteer to work Christmas and most other family-focused holidays. I figure there's no point in me being at home alone with a glass of wine when someone with kids at home could be watching them open their gifts. I don't mind volunteering, but sometimes I feel that I'm being taken advantage of just because I don't have kids. I have mixed feelings about it. Sure, I can work and even get extra pay because it's a holiday, but I also can't help but realize how alone I am while my coworkers are at home by the fire having a cozy family time."

The holidays were a challenge this past year for Renee, because her husband David died in December after a long battle with cancer. She shared, "My husband died on December 15th. His adult children were here for a little over a week before he died, and two of the three stayed the rest of the second week until the funeral. His older son and his family spent Christmas with me. We went to church on Christmas Eve, and the next day we had a very low-key Christmas dinner. My husband was cremated on New Year's Eve, and afterwards, we went out for a nice lunch to celebrate his life. Then the holidays were over, and I was here alone."

While listening to Renee share her holiday experience and talk about her husband's death, I realized that she may have wondered if these adult children from her spouse's first marriage would begin to drift out of her life now that their father had gone. This possibility has likely brought up more emotion for her because she's been reminded of the child that she chose not to have.

Roger the financial analyst shared, "All holidays are hard because they bring up those feelings of wanting family." His wife Annie added, "I've tried to find opportunities to create my own sense of family. For example, there was a woman, Trudy, who worked in my office for many years who had one son with whom she really had no relationship. We kept in touch after her retirement, and she finally ended up in a nursing home. Trudy had many friends who spent many hours with her and were much more like family than her own son was."

QUESTIONS TO CONSIDER

How did you spend your last holiday season?

If you don't have family nearby, how do you feel a sense of closeness on family-focused holidays?

Mother's Day/Father's Day

Every year, huge amounts of energy are put into celebrating Mother's Day and Father's Day, sending out a strong message that parents are greatly valued in our culture. According to the National Retail Foundation, Mother's Day is a 14-billion-dollar industry. According to Mother's Day Central, restaurants in the United States claim that it's their busiest day of the entire year! Most childfree adults view these days as playful or simply as Hallmark Holidays. Diane admitted, "Those parent-specific holidays really don't have any impact on us other than the *obligation* to our own parents." Renee agreed, saying, "I've always felt that Mother's and Father's Days are sort of made up!"

Mother's Day is a 14-billion-dollar industry.

Denise has no sadness about not being recognized on Mother's Day. She said, "I love special holidays like Mother's Day and Father's Day. I celebrate my sisters on these days, and I always send my childfree sister in New York a card "from her cat." Just because I'm not a mother doesn't mean I can't celebrate those who are."

When I asked Carrie about Mother's Day, she shrugged and said, "Kids are so selfish that you don't get much attention or recognition anyway until they've had children of their own. Even then, it might not happen."

Mark shared that it has never occurred to him that he might be somehow missing out on Father's Day. His wife, Sarah, gets cards from her nieces and nephews on Mother's Day, and they enjoy doing something special for Mark's mom.

Tracy suggested, "People put too many expectations on the day", echoing the sentiment of many of the other respondents that it's more of a Hallmark Holiday than anything else.

I was surprised to hear that none of these childfree adults felt left out or sad on these special parent days. I wonder how different the responses would have been if I'd met with more adults who yearned to have children but were unable to do so for whatever reason. How might such a person cope with parent-focused days when not having children is a source of sadness for them? One woman described her experience in her blog, in which she shared,

"Often Mother's Day is a day I hide under the covers in bed, afraid of the sadness I'd face if I left the house."

"In the nine years of knowing of my infertility, I think I've made it to church on Mother's Day maybe twice. I remember watching as the mothers got roses. It felt so painful that there was a visual marker of how broken my womanhood is, that I can't just pop out a kid like all these other women. Often Mother's Day is a day I hide under the covers in bed, afraid of the sadness I'd face if I left the house."

I've often thought that there should be a day recognizing child-free adults. When I asked Arno about this, he commented, "Perhaps we should be recognized and thanked for not contributing to the demise of the environment."

Author Cara Swann discusses this topic in her 2001 article, "World Childfree Day." She writes:

Admit it, the title probably made you curious if such a day was honored. And as yet, I have to say it hasn't been suggested OR slated for a worldwide celebration—but why not? As a childfree person, I keep wondering if we'll ever be a large enough group to get recognition for OUR contribution to society in remaining childfree? I suppose what had me thinking along these lines is that we've just celebrated Mother's Day, and soon Father's Day will come around. And while we all have parents to honor, perhaps some of us feel left out when these time-honored dates occur. In truth, I've certainly witnessed some biological parents who have been so inadequate (or downright abusive/neglectful) in these roles they have no right to be "honored." Others though do deserve the recognition for lifetime devotion and dedication it takes to be good parents.

But what of those of us who have no children by choice? As many of my previous columns have pointed out, the childfree make many worthwhile contributions to society—not only by NOT contributing to worldwide overpopulation, but also by using their time as productive members of communities in work-related and volunteer capacities.

As the world increasingly groans under the overwhelming weight of too many human beings, we hear nothing but dire news from politicians about the problems, and ridiculous rhetoric about "maintaining the status quo" regardless of how we have to damage the earth's environment to do so. Our energy supply is becoming inadequate, gas prices soar, gridlock on the metropolitan highways, and yet no politician dares speak about the one aspect that would help curb these growing problems: Limit the population by incentives not to reproduce.

"Perhaps we should be recognized and thanked for not contributing to the demise of the environment."

So I think we childfree should consider creating our own worldwide day of recognition. I can just imagine the antagonism this would garner from the childed, but it could be a way to spread our message: Not everyone has to reproduce. Happiness can be found without having children. And possibly most important, we leave no offspring to add to the world's growing population who are depleting earth's resources at an alarming rate.[14]

Creating Balance

This chapter describes the stories of childfree adults who appear to be living balanced lives. They all had or took the time to participate in this project, which speaks to at least some degree of flexibility in their schedules. This, of course, is not the case for all childfree adults. In my psychology practice, a common complaint I hear from patients has to do with a lack of balance in their daily lives. I define balance as the ability to make time for fun, work, rest, relationships, creativity, spirituality, healthy eating, and exercise. While those who are parents most often express a lack of balance, adults without children are also susceptible. Our imbalance typically stems from being too focused on work or extracurricular activities. The single childfree adult may feel financial pressures that lead them to take on extra work, or, as Nicole described earlier in this chapter, they may be pressured into working overtime because they lack family obligations. The childfree adult may be expected to take on more responsibility in caring for elderly parents because they appear to have more free time than their siblings with children. When patients tell me that these kinds of situations have resulted in anxiety or depression, I encourage them to examine their lifestyles and look for ways to make concrete changes.

Mike, a childfree banker, exemplifies this perfectly. When Mike and I met, he shared that he'd recently turned fifty, had never been married, did not date, and had devoted himself to his career. Mike's physician had referred him to me because he'd had a panic attack at work; initially he thought he was having a heart attack, but his doctor checked him out and told him that it was just stress. Mike told me he had not been able to sleep well for several months. He was irritable and short with his staff at work. When I asked for more information on his daily life, Mike relayed that he typically worked seventy hours a week at the bank, plus he kept in touch by email and cell phone from home. He took care of after-hour tasks so that his colleagues with families would not be burdened. He didn't exercise and he had no social life. He added that gradually over the years, all his friends had married and started families, and he'd filled the gap in his life by throwing himself more and more into his job. He typically slept for fewer than five hours a night, finding himself tossing and turning even on nights when he tried to turn in early. After he told me his story, I couldn't help but respond, "Wow, it's no wonder you're anxious!" This comment brought a slight smile to his face.

I told Mike that his panic attacks had likely been caused by overwork and general lack of balance in his life. He worked with me over the next six months to make concrete changes, starting with working with his colleagues on creating a more equitable way to handle after-hours tasks and therefore limiting his work hours. He started to exercise and to get in touch with old friends. Mike's anxiety and depression dissipated within two months, and he left therapy shortly thereafter.

I know from my own experience what happens when life balance is lost. A few years ago, I was routinely putting sixty or more hours a week into my practice. Because I didn't have a family at home, I had trouble saying no to clients who requested evening or weekend sessions. I wasn't immediately aware of any problems, but before too long I began to have trouble sleeping. Though I'd never had insomnia in the past, my new pattern was to fall asleep easily but then to wake up in the middle of the night and be unable to fall back to sleep for several hours. I tend to be stubborn, so I resisted making changes for several years. I treated my insomnia with herbal remedies and exercise. As my fortieth birthday drew near, I suddenly became aware that I was *way* out of balance. I began to cut back my work hours and I tried to "slow down." I devoted more time to pleasurable hobbies, friendships, and just doing nothing. Almost immediately, my sleeping patterns normalized. I remind myself often that not having children means I have more time in my life for leisure pursuits, and that my time for these activities is worth protecting. It has gradually gotten easier for me to maintain my boundaries and to treat my personal leisure time as equally valuable to productive time at the office.

Each of us has personalized warning signs that tell us when we're out of balance in our daily lives. For me, it's waking up at 2 am and being unable to fall right back to sleep; this is a sure sign that I've been overextending in one area or another and that I'm out of balance. When this happens, I renew my commitment to sticking with my set working hours, and I remind myself of the value of my time away from work.

> **Parents with two children put in 7.5 hours a day raising them, which adds up to 57,661 hours over eighteen years.**

Each of my patients has his or her own unique signals, including increased cravings for certain foods or alcohol, physical symptoms such as headaches or GI distress, an inability to concentrate, irritability, depression, panic attacks, or trouble with turning off worrisome thoughts. Once you realize that having a balanced life is a *must*, you are much more capable of setting firm boundaries that allow you to maintain a healthy day-to-day existence over time.

QUESTIONS TO CONSIDER

What are your personal signs of imbalance?

How do you get yourself back on track when you notice that you're out of balance?

Parenting Takes a Lot of Time!

"My husband and I affirmatively chose not to have chil-
dren, so we could devote ourselves to our beloved work,
extensive worldwide travel, our favorite pastimes, friends
and family. We have a lifestyle most of our married-with-
children friends can only dream about. And it's one we could
only have dreamed about, too, if we had had children."

—Bonnie Erbe, PBS commentator and columnist

Many childfree adults struggle to maintain balance in their lives, but this is even more of a challenge for parents. I recently stumbled across a fascinating article that took a look at time spent on child rearing. According to author Susan Lang, time-use experts from Cornell University found that parents with two children put in 7.5 hours a day raising them—three times more than experts had previously estimated.[15] These researchers added all the hours parents put into raising their kids, including primary child care tasks such as bathing, dressing, teaching, supervising, counseling, driving, and feeding children, as well as secondary child care activities such as cooking, housework, and hobbies. They also included shared leisure, household work, and mealtime. According to my calculations, 7.5 hours a day for eighteen years adds up to 57,661 hours.

Of course people might argue that during many of the hours parents spend with their children, they do things that would be done even if the kids weren't around, like cooking and eating meals. The qualitative difference is that when a childfree adult does these activities, they are focused on their own needs or those of their partner; when a parent performs these tasks, their child is typically center stage. Parents frequently choose to prepare foods that will please their child, and dinnertime conversation is often focused on what the child did that day or what his or her plans are for the next.

Even if a parent finds raising children to be enjoyable, it's still is a huge commitment that results in the sacrifice of other activities.

Compare this time commitment to a PhD dissertation. My dissertation required about eighteen hours a week for a year, or 1,000 hours total. People are often impressed with my accomplishment, but compared to the time spent on raising a child, writing a dissertation is nothing! These days, I prefer to saunter rather than dash through my hours away from work. This shift is happening for me at a time when many of my same-age peers with children are constantly on the go—they never have enough hours in the day to get everything accomplished. Most of our friends are older, and if they have children they're well settled into the empty-nest phase of their lives. I gravitate toward them because they have time for me!

Childfree adults are more likely to have an easier time keeping or regaining balance in life, simply because there are no time demands to raise children. Keeping an ongoing awareness of your own personal signals that suggest balance has been lost is an easy way to stay on track.

The common thread for the childfree adults I interviewed is that they truly relish their leisure time. Whether or not they're coupled up, evenings and weekends are a time for relaxing and rejuvenating, and are not just for doing chores. According to the aforementioned Cornell University study, a childfree adult has almost eight hours more free time a day than a parent with two children. Of course, there are some childfree adults who are overextended and out of balance in their lives, but for these individuals, reclaiming balance is an attainable goal that involves establishing healthy boundaries in their lives. This is not so easy for parents when the time-consumer is their own children. I expected to hear some stories of childfree adults who feel bored or lonely in the evening when they imagine parents are at home with their children focused on homework, dinner, and laundry—but this was not the case. All the people I interviewed have had many years—basically their entire adult life—to figure out how to spend their evening time, and the benefits people expressed were numerous.

Perhaps the take-away message here is that the opportunity to do whatever you want with your evenings and weekends is a gift, and this opportunity is something that many people at middle age and beyond rarely experience. We ought to relish this and not take it for granted.

In the words of Joan Baez, "You don't get to choose how you're going to die. Or when. You can only decide how you're going to live. Now."

QUESTIONS TO CONSIDER

When you examine the ingredients of your week, including time for rest, exercise, healthy eating, relationships, spirituality, work, play, and creativity, are you in balance?

Do you feel that your friends with children have more difficulty maintaining balance in their lives than you do?

What makes the difference?

Are you getting what you want from your free time?

If not, what changes might you make to increase your satisfaction?

What are your favorite times of the day?

Are holidays and other special times, including vacations, stressful for you?

What changes could you make in the way you handle these special occasions that would make them more enjoyable?

CHAPTER 5
LOVE AND FRIENDSHIP

"My partner and I don't have kids, and so our quality of life is fluid and spontaneous. Not having children doesn't pressure us to work on our relationship. In fact, it's the opposite. My friends with children put energy into their relationship to keep it strong for the sake of the kids. We don't have to put in the energy because it's just there."

—Elizabeth, age forty-eight

It's no secret that couples and singles without kids have quite different lives than those who are parents. Most of us have more leisure time and discretionary income, as well as the ability to pack up and go at a moment's notice. Childfree couples have more time to spend together. And yet, despite these freedoms, childfree adults face unique relationship challenges, with both our romantic partners and our friends. And when a childfree adult becomes involved with someone who has kids, an entirely different set of complications arises.

Childfree Couples

If one of my peers who is busy raising a family were to peek into my life for a moment, she might very well view me as selfish, because I have the luxury of spending huge amounts of time with Chris, and because I pursue my own interests. On a typical weekday, Chris and

I enjoy having our meals together at home, and on the weekends we go out for long bicycle rides, see movies, and have get-togethers with friends. It's not uncommon for us to bail on the to-do list because it's just the two of us, and no one's going to be harmed by putting off those tasks for another week.

Typical couples start out by focusing most of their time on one another, but this togetherness comes to an abrupt halt when the first child arrives. Their lives change, and it's not uncommon for their time together to decrease significantly. After all, as I mentioned in chapter 4, it takes an average of 7.5 hours a day to raise two children to the age of eighteen. Although there are many households in which both parents work outside of the home, one recent trend is to keep the children out of day care. This involves parents working opposing shifts and caring separately for the little ones at home. This scenario often results in partners passing one another like ships in the night, with very limited time to be together as a couple or a family. One essay in Lori Leibovich's book, *Maybe Baby*, tells the story of a husband and wife who go out to the same movie at separate times and later meet up at home to talk about the film. This couple goes to extraordinary lengths to have shared experiences despite the scheduling restraints caused by having a child, but it's just not the same as going to the movie together.

For such couples, because their relationship gets put on the back burner during the child-rearing years, it's often found that they have little in common once the kids begin to grow up. Child-free couples do not experience these kinds of abrupt transitions, as they have a relationship evolution that is much more fluid and allows for natural growth together, or natural moving apart. There's no obligation to stay together for the sake of children, and it's easier to grow together simply due to a greater abundance of time and the opportunity to continue to participate in the shared interests that brought them together in the first place. One of the childfree adults I interviewed described this situation with her partner. Elizabeth, the marketing consultant who lives in an urban condominium with her partner Maria, shared, "Since Maria and I don't have children, our quality of life is fluid and spontaneous. Not having children doesn't pressure us to work on our relationship. In fact, it's the opposite. My friends with children put energy into their relationship to keep it strong for the sake of the kids. Maria and I don't have to put in the energy, because it's just there."

Reflecting on Elizabeth's words, I realized that Chris's and my experience has been very similar. We were initially drawn to each other because of our common interests—we're both psychologists, athletes, and conversationalists—and because of these commonalities, we tend to spend most of our leisure time together

> "Our life has focused on our relationship and our individual interests rather than on starting a family."

simply because we want to. Our mealtime discussions are generally focused on psychology, our joint sporting activities, and current events. If we had a child, dinnertime conversations would undoubtedly be dominated by subjects like diapers and babysitters; we'd also find ourselves monitoring what we said in front of the child. If this pattern were to continue over a couple of decades, we would forget how to flirt with one another and how to talk about those topics that once brought us together. This pattern certainly explains why so many couples you see in restaurants sit through their entire meals in silence. They've forgotten how to talk to one another in an authentic way, and they've forgotten about the things they used to enjoy discussing in the years before the children arrived.

Suzanne the legal secretary told me, "From the start of our time together, John and I agreed that having kids was not for us, and so our life has focused on our relationship and our individual interests rather than on starting a family. Our relationship has always been mutually nourishing and healthy and we have strived both individually and together to be more enriched people. I've noticed that couples with children often don't have the extra energy to put into their relationship for the sheer time and effort that it takes to raise kids."

Another couple with many years together is Laurie and Craig, both in their early forties. Laurie shared, "I found the perfect mate at an early age. Craig and I have both always known that we didn't want children. Our relationship is very strong. We have lots of opportunity to spend time together uninterrupted and to act spontaneously. This keeps things fresh and exciting. Some people seem to stay married 'for the kids' and for no other compelling reason. It's sad to see people who are not happy in their relationship but aren't motivated to get out of it and start living their lives again. Marriage is two people; couples should want to be married to their partner, not to the family unit."

Marital quality often drops after the transition to parenthood, and there is an increase in marital happiness after the children leave home.

Thinking about Laurie's comments on couples staying together for the sake of the kids compelled me to take a look at the research that's been done on the impact of children on marital satisfaction. In a 2009 *New York Times* article, Stephanie Coontz, professor of history at Evergreen College in Olympia, Washington, cited two decades of research which concluded that marital quality often drops after the transition to parenthood, and that there is an increase in marital happiness after the children leave home.[16] A closer look at this phenomenon showed that the average drop in marital satisfaction was almost entirely accounted for by the couples who slip into, disagree over, or are ambivalent about being parents. Couples who planned or equally welcomed the conception were likely to maintain or to even increase their marital satisfaction after the birth of the child. So, an important component of relationship satisfaction is the agreement by both partners on whether or not to have kids.

It's a similar scenario with childfree couples—if both partners agree fully that having children is not for them, then their individual happiness ought to be fairly high, but if one wants children and the other resists, there will be tension in the marriage.

Coontz also noted that marital quality tends to decline for both partners when they shift into more traditional gender roles, such as the wife leaving her job and the husband working more. Finally, she found that marital satisfaction drops when couples become so involved in parenting that they pay less attention to each other. The time people spend with their children is actually on the rise—according to Coontz, married mothers spent 20 percent more time with their children in 2000 than they did in 1965, and married fathers spent more than twice as much time with their kids. It all adds up to less time together as a couple, focused on one another.

Some might argue that couples with kids have a lot to talk over, including child rearing and financial decisions. A few of the childfree couples I interviewed expressed concern that, while not especially fun, having so many child-focused topics to discuss and decide on might actually strengthen a relationship. Mark, the engineer in his mid-fifties, stated, "I wonder if childfree couples might have greater relationship stress since rearing children is not a central reason to be together. There is a challenging balance between togetherness and separateness that may not be as edgy if, as a couple, you're focused on growing a family."

This sentiment was echoed by Jill, the network engineer. "I see my couple friends with young kids talking more fondly about their life at home than the rest of us. As I think about it, though, I remember that it's about their interactions with their kids and with their spouses as the parents of their kids. I don't hear a lot about their actual adult relationships with each other." This indeed would seem to be the case more often than not—that while parents are talking with one another, they aren't chatting the way they did before the children were born, about those common interests that brought them together in the first place.

All in all, though, childfree couples are quick to say that not having kids has impacted their relationships in a positive way. Diane the accountant shared, "I believe Patrick and I have a more relaxed relationship without children. Our friends seem to be constantly running around taking their children to one event after another. I actually believe couples with children have to put more effort into their relationship to keep things from being 'all about the kids.'

> "Our friends seem to be constantly running around taking their children to one event after another."

Finding time alone or having a date night becomes even more critical when you have kids. If anything, I think we have more time to work on our relationship since we don't have to focus on the needs of children before our own. Patrick and I lead a pretty quiet lifestyle—we love our dogs, enjoy movies, dining out, plays, musicals, concerts, and riding our motorcycles. I think our lives would be drastically different if we had children. Right now we never have to think about anyone but ourselves. We recognize the selfishness in that statement, but we really enjoy our life and what it has become. Our social life is quite different from our friends with children, as most of their social activities revolve around their children, such as a trip to the zoo instead of a night out dancing in Seattle. Our friends have tended to come and go in and out of our lives depending on our circumstances, and that's okay, because it's our relationship that is the constant."

Although the childfree couples I have interviewed all seem to have strong, healthy marriages, divorce is still prevalent in the childfree community. The divorce rate among childfree couples is, however, only slightly higher than among couples with children. Couples with children often feel compelled to stay together for the sake of the kids, but this statistic shows the possibility that childfree couples are just as deeply attached to aspects of their relationships. In my clinical practice, I continue to have men and women in my office who express great unhappiness in their marriages. Often they're contemplating leaving their spouse. Many are parents, and they claim their children are the primary reason for staying in their marriage. Even after the children are grown and out of the house, there is hesitance to leave because of grandchildren, holiday gatherings, and myriad other attachments to one another that would not exist without the kids. I also talk to partners in childfree marriages who express hesitance to leave due to their emotional and financial dependence on one another, their combined social networks, and their concerns over who will get the family pets. These couples report having as strong a sense of family as those with children, and in many ways they are more emotionally attached and dependent on one another as couples with children, because it's just the two of them.

QUESTIONS TO CONSIDER

Do you feel that your partnership is stronger because you do not have children?

Have you and your partner been in agreement on the decision regarding whether or not to have kids? If not, how has this impacted your relationship?

Have you considered leaving your partner because of disagreements about whether or not to have children? What factors caused you to hesitate?

Childfree Singles

Childfree singles face their own unique set of problems. A common complaint involves difficulty connecting with the opposite sex. FBI agent Nicole is tall, dark-haired, and in her mid-thirties. She shared, "Not wanting to have children has significantly affected my dating life. I've been dumped by men who knew from the start that I didn't want children, but thought they could change my mind when they were ready to start a family. I've also dated men with children who didn't want to 'hold me back' because of their having so many restrictions and obligations to their kids. I've also found that men paying child support are less likely to splurge for a weekend getaway or even a night out. Most of the time, I wind up paying for half, if not all, of the 'fun' expenses. I haven't had a serious relationship with someone with kids, so I typically don't get involved in their financial dealings. It's frustrating, though, when guys I've dated casually disappeared during holidays because their children always come first. And then there's the general lack of commitment when things get tough. Two of my friends tell me that if they didn't have children with their spouse they would leave today. I find that my relationships tend to end without someone trying to work things out—there is nothing binding me to that other person so there's no reason to put a lot of extra time and/ or energy into keeping a relationship together once it hits a rough patch."

> "Not wanting to have children has significantly affected my dating life. I've been dumped by men who knew from the start that I didn't want children, but thought they could change my mind when they were ready to start a family."

Nicole shared that she had two dinner dates this past week, one with a man who shares custody of his 7-year-old daughter and one with another man who's childfree and ten years younger than her. She had to arrange times and dates around the first man's ex-wife's work schedule so he would have a free evening to get together. The other called her out of the blue and they met for dinner an hour later. "It gets old trying to work around my schedule, their schedule, and their ex-wife's schedule just to find time to get together. After a while, I feel begin to think, *Why bother?*, and I sense this attitude in the men as well. It's also hard to never be someone's first priority. Your kids should always come first, but it's difficult to accept that when someone is constantly canceling or changing plans because something with the kids came up."

Working in a male-dominated profession, Nicole has found herself surrounded for the most part by men who are either married or are divorced but still raising children. At thirty-seven, she's at an awkward age to be seeking a partner who, like herself, has no children. I imagine that if I were to approach Nicole ten years from now, when she is forty-seven, she would report that these same men are more available with their time, emotion, and money, simply because their children have left the nest.

"I made a personal decision not to date anyone with children, and I considered kids to be a red flag. This was simply not the lifestyle I wanted for myself or for my future."

Elizabeth, the marketing consultant from Boston, told me that she avoided this particular problem by not getting involved with women who have children. She shared, "I made a personal decision not to date anyone with children, and I considered kids to be a red flag. This was simply not the lifestyle I wanted for myself or for my future." In the pool of available lesbian women and gay men, there is a much larger percentage who are childfree than in the heterosexual population, so there are more opportunities to meet partners who do not have kids.

Tracy, the web designer, talked about her frustrations with being single in a couple's world. "I've noticed that people have couples, not singles, over for dinner. One of my friends finally got involved with someone over the last year, and she told me that she gets invited to more gatherings now that she has a partner. We've discussed this, and decided that women in relationships don't want to be around single women because they see what their life would be like if they were single. They may also feel some threat from a single woman because people assume that a single woman is on the make."

Other childfree singles avoid dating altogether. Denise, the psychiatric office manager in her early sixties, hasn't been involved in a romantic relationship since her divorce over twenty years ago. "Part of this choice has been that I didn't want to deal with the trials and tribulations of someone else's children. If I had partnered up with someone after my divorce, he would almost certainly have had kids, just given the statistical chances. My friends who have married men with children have difficult times, regardless of the ages of the children. I think that children of divorce face unique challenges, and I didn't want to burden myself with those kinds of issues."

For childfree adults who are clearly frustrated by their lack of progress in dating and would like to connect with others who, like themselves, don't have and don't want to have kids, a dating web site—aptly named IDoNotWantKids.com—has been created to help. It very well may be that, as the number of childfree adults grows, we begin to resemble other unique groups, such as smokers, who are often frowned on by general society and therefore tend to stick together.

QUESTIONS TO CONSIDER

If you're a childfree single, has it been difficult to find appropriate dating partners?

Would you consider limiting your dating to other childfree adults exclusively? What advantages and disadvantages would there be in doing so?

Childfree Adults as Stepparents

Many childfree adults end up, at some point, in a relationship with someone who has kids. If these adults never wanted to be a parent, this could be stressful for everyone concerned. I remember a client I worked with a couple of years ago, a woman I'll call Heidi. She had two teenage daughters from a previous marriage and was living with a childfree woman her own age. They had none of the common issues about the former spouse, but they frequently argued about Heidi's children. The childfree partner wanted more of Heidi's time and attention, and she also was unhappy about the amount of money being spent on the children. The partner was in a very different financial position than Heidi, having worked all her life without children to support, so she was thinking about leaving her job to explore other career options. Heidi felt resentment toward her partner for having so many options, and they clearly had not worked out a financial arrangement that would move them toward a partnership together. In a situation like this, it's complicated to find a solution that feels fair to both partners. Often the person without kids has worked hard and saved without the distraction of child rearing. The partner with children is usually just trying to get by month to month, both in terms of finances and daily tasks, and she may look at her childfree partner with some resentment. A strong commitment is needed to keep a couple with these significant life discrepancies together in the long haul, and many choose to separate because of the challenge.

Some childfree adults report that they never really bond to their partner's children but instead relate to them only when it's necessary to do so. I asked Carrie, the medical biller, about her role as a stepmom to her husband Steven's kids. She shared, "They only came to visit for a couple of weeks each summer, and I loved having them for a few days but was always glad to see them go. I enjoyed cooking for them and taking care of them, but I didn't really enjoy sitting down at the table and interacting with them."

I have coped with the addition of Chris's grown children to my life in a different way. It's been helpful for me to stay far away from a maternal role with them and to treat them like any young adult I might meet, as if they were the grown children of a friend. I work hard to find fun things to talk to them about, and I indulge them with special treats from time to time, but I don't give advice unless it's asked for. In our time together, Chris and I have avoided conflict about finances by keeping our money separate, and we've accepted the fact that, because he has children and I don't, we are in different places in terms of our financial responsibility and how much we've been able to prepare for our future.

QUESTIONS TO CONSIDER

Is it reasonable to avoid involvement with someone who has children simply to avoid complications?

If you're involved with a partner who has kids, how have you managed to deal with the inherent complications?

Friendships

Until I reached my mid-thirties, I was a member of an elite group of childfree adults with whom I'd been friends for years. By the time we reached our late thirties, I anticipated we'd all remain childfree. It came as quite a surprise when two of the five announced that they were expecting within the same year. It was particularly unexpected because we were all established in our careers and settled into relationships, and none of us seemed to be headed in the direction of having kids. The subject of children seldom came up. It just seemed to me that we were all busy having fun and that this would continue until we were old and gray. I felt good about my own decision not to have a child, knowing that I wouldn't be alone, and when the occasional twinge of babylust hit me, it faded away almost as quickly as it appeared. When my friend Linda called me with the news that she was pregnant, I tried to show her I was happy, but in reality I felt a huge wave of sadness as I anticipated that our friendship was about to undergo a permanent change. Because we live on opposite ends of the country, I wasn't part of her pregnancy experience. I remember her calling with complaints of plantar fasciitis that made it tough to do her job as a nurse. When the baby came, I sent flowers—a huge bouquet of lavender carnations. I remember feeling a combination of envy that I wasn't a new mother and relief that all I had to do was get online and choose flowers. I went to visit Linda a few weeks later, and by the end of the weekend, it was clear to me that our friendship would never be quite the same. Linda was now a mother and her focus had shifted from her own goals to what was best for her child. Of course I realized that this was healthy and normal, and it was even what I would want for Linda and her son, but there was a loss for me.

Later that year, I had the same reaction to the news from another old friend, Thomas, that his wife was expecting their first child. Once his son arrived, the child naturally became the center of Thomas's life. Through the years, Linda and Thomas have held their children as the top priority in their lives, and this is where they've put most of their emotional energy. Our group of friends, myself included, has had a strong sense of being put on the back burner. As their lives have become more complicated by the demands of parenthood, Linda and Thomas have disappeared at times from the radar screen for months on end. At a point where I've been spending more and more time examining who I am and where I want to take my life, they are becoming more and more involved in the lives of their children. Last December, I opened Thomas's holiday card to find a page filled with photographs of his son and copious information on the child's accomplishments from the past year. I wondered where Thomas had gone—it was almost as if he, himself, was shrinking over time. I often find myself asking Linda and Thomas what grade their boys are in, and I selfishly look forward to the day when the boys will graduate from high school and they will once again have time to have fun with me.

Some of the childfree adults I met also had strong feelings about how the arrival of kids has impacted their friendships. Suzanne, the legal secretary in her mid-thirties, said, "Just a couple of years ago we had a much larger circle of friends, but because several of the couples had children, John and I took a leave of absence from the group. If we had been long-time friends, we would have continued to socialize with them as normal, but because they were relatively new friends, socializing became awkward. I felt predominantly left out. They were all new parents and simply had more to talk about with each other, and perhaps more of an interest to go on outings with other parents. Although it was awkward, and in many ways painful, this seemed totally natural and necessary to me. I have to admit, however, that I have a fear that some of our dearest friends will decide to have kids and then things just won't be the same. They, too, will have crossed over to the other side." Suzanne shared that because she and John are unable to count on their friends to be there for them in the long run, they have become more dependent on one another. "Our friends are absolutely important to us, but they aren't 'number one.' I do, however, feel a special kinship with our childless friends, like we're in some special club. We look at each other and say things like, 'We childless people need to stick together!' A part of me hopes that we'll all be there for each other when we're old, so that no one is left alone."

> "I have a fear that one of our dearest couple friends will decide to have kids and then things just won't be the same. They, too, will have crossed over to the other side."

When your friends start to have children, it's time to decide whether to join right in with the child-rearing experience or to accept the fact that the friendship is going to change. Annie, who's in her mid-thirties, shared her experience of observing the busy lives of her friends who are parents, noting, "My friend, Karen, said that it would be great to have just one hour a week to go to the gym by herself." If Karen doesn't even have the time to go to the gym, where is she finding time to spend with Annie? It's easy to see why so many friendships fall apart once children are born, simply due to lack of time together. Nicole expressed her frustration that she can't find friends who are available to travel with her because everyone her own age is busy raising their families.

Other childfree adults complained that their friends with kids delegate when social events will be scheduled. Jackie the paralegal ranted, "People should put their children first, but you have to have a balance. Your children have to see that you are a person and respect you as a person. I've had numerous occasions when friends have changed plans that they've had with me due to things going on with their kids. It's okay if this happens once or twice, but if it happens more than that, I tend to give up on the friendship. I'm involved in a group of other office managers who get together for social gatherings. The schedule always has to revolve around the two women who have children. Somehow that just doesn't seem fair."

It's also not unusual for childfree adults to report feeling left out or like a misfit in a group. Just recently, Chris and I hosted a party in our home. There were several occasions during the party when I initiated conversations with some of the other women there, and they began to talk about their children or grandchildren right away. I realized that we had little in common, and, as is common for me, I gravitated toward the men, who were more likely to be discussing business or politics. After everyone left, I pulled out the guest list to see who hadn't shown up, and it hit me—out of a group of twenty-five men and women, there was only one other child-free adult besides me. I was shocked by how much of an anomaly I really am. I have not experienced so many things that parents take for granted, including changing hundreds if not thousands of diapers, getting a child off to his first day of school, saving for a college fund, leaving work early to go to a soccer game, having family-focused vacations as opposed to couple weekends away, and looking ahead to grandchildren. Sometimes not having these things to talk about with other adults results in awkward silence, and at times I feel a sense of embarrassment and find myself thinking that they must wonder why I never grew up and joined the adult world. In these moments, I sometimes ask myself why I didn't simply choose the more common path in life and why I decided to do things my own way—a way that resulted in me feeling alone in a crowd, like a misfit.

> "Out of a group of twenty-five men and women, there was only one other childfree adult besides me."

Perhaps in order to avoid these kind of dead-end conversations and to feel okay about our choices, many childfree adults have started to join together to socialize. In Seattle, there is a meet-up group just for childfree couples that plans frequent social gatherings throughout the city. NoKidding.net is a social networking organization with groups all over the world that was formed to bring together childfree adults. The social lives and interests of parents tend to be quite different from childfree adults. Chris and I know a lot of folks who have children, but none of them invite us to their homes. They must think that we wouldn't want to be around their kids, which is true in most cases. Likewise, we never invite children to our home, and if someone with a child is coming, I make it quite clear that it will be an adult-focused gathering. In talking to other childfree adults, I discovered that many of them also prefer adult-only gatherings. Laurie, the engineer, noted, "Our social lives are mostly related to sports, cars, and work acquaintances. We are active within our motorcycle club and have met a number of close friends through motorcycle riding. We like to camp and ride motorcycles, both off-road and street bikes. I play soccer and snowboard and have made many friends through those activities. Craig is really into cars and has a lot of friends that he connects with over working on and/or racing cars. We both enjoy hiking with friends and family. In our twenties and thirties, the majority of friends we spent most of our time with had no children. Now, in our forties, we're also spending time with friends who have adult children. It was a choice not to hang out with people with young kids. This may have limited us, but it worked out just fine and kept us sane. We live our lives on our own terms and don't have to make time or room for other people's kids."

Other childfree adults, including singles, have found ways to have full social lives. Denise, the psychiatric office manager, shared, "I feel that my social life is rich. I live alone, but I have many friends. I have one friend who I have dinner with every Friday night. She's also single and lives alone, so we take the time to review our weeks with each other, like a partnered person would do at home each night. I've been in a book club for twenty years, and I'm on a couple of boards. Not having a family of my own has meant that I have more time to give to the community and also to be involved in things that I enjoy."

Denise told me, "If I'd had children, I probably would have initially made friends with the mothers of kids in the same school or other activities, but those friendships would not have endured the test of time unless we had shared interests and activities. My friendships with women I met before they had kids have persisted, even though they have had children. Of course, my social life is a bit different from those friends in that they get together with other parents and have playgroups with their kids. Their lives may be more child-centered than mine, although when I get together with friends with small kids, the activities tend to be child-centered anyway, and I don't mind that. I'm certainly able to be more flexible than people with children, and I frequently make social plans with friends with little kids based on *their* schedules. Over time, I've recognized that I've needed to reach out more for social connections than my married friends with children. Taking a child to a soccer game is an immediate social connection with parents of other players. For me, I need to contact someone and make a plan to get together."

Denise has clearly thrived in her friendships, perhaps due to her outgoing, nurturing personality, and because she is organized and tends to plan ahead. A childfree adult who is more reserved or introverted and who tends to live spontaneously would be more likely to feel lonely and to be socially isolated.

Carrie, the medical biller, also described how being childfree has impacted her friendships over the years. She shared, "My best friend has three children, but they're grown up now. Through the decades my friendships changed. I would hang out with younger people or folks who had already raised kids. Steven and I didn't really interact with friends with their children. We intentionally planned adult activities, and when our friends with kids got together with us, they saw this as an opportunity to get away from the children."

QUESTIONS TO CONSIDER

How have your friendships changed over time as a result of your friends becoming parents?

What have you done to ensure that you've remained socially connected and not felt lonely?

Support Networks

A unique problem for adults without kids is the potential lack of a strong support network. In our busy lives, people rush around focused on their own business, and they often don't have the time or energy to add someone outside of their immediate family to their list of people for whom to be responsible. Because women in general are more prone than men to develop close and nurturing friendships, childfree women are more likely than childfree men to have a tight network of friends and colleagues who can help out in an emergency. Denise told me about her experience two years ago when she broke her leg and was unable to drive or get out for a couple of weeks. "My girlfriends got together and planned my life. They set up a schedule and told me who would be driving me from day to day and who would be dropping meals off at my apartment. It was amazing and I felt truly blessed!" I heard a dramatically different story from Walt, a fifty-year-old sales consultant from Georgia, who shared, "Last year I fell off of a ladder while working around my house, and I broke my back. It was a terrible time for me. I could hardly move for several weeks and the only folks who stepped in to help were my secretary and one neighbor. At times like those, you realize who your real friends are—what I found out is that I don't have many."

When I asked Arno about his friendships and whether they were stronger because he did not have children, he noted, "I've never really thought about needing to develop close friendships because of not having kids, because let's face it, everyone ultimately dies alone. I don't have much of a social life. Coming to this coffee shop to meet you is the first time I've been out to a place other than to a store in almost six months. Even if I'd become a dad, I wouldn't have been a soccer dad; my children would have suffered. I was too selfish and too reclusive to be a father." At this point in his life,

Arno is able to take care of himself and to live independently. He's married, but I couldn't help but wonder what would happen to him if he were to suffer an accident, like Walt, that left him in need of help. If his wife were not available to help out, he clearly would not have a supportive network of friends who would rush over to drive him to the doctor or to make meals for him.

Other childfree adults, even those in relationships, also talked about feeling vulnerable. Suzanne noted that her biggest concern about old age is having to live without her husband, John. She explained, "I worry about what will happen if John dies before I do, because we are so far from our families and we've moved around quite a bit and don't have extremely close friends. I still have a strong family network and I think I'll get back into that if need be in the future. I don't worry about not having money, but I worry about my health and not being able to take care of myself, being in an old folk's home and alone and miserable." While reflecting on Suzanne's words, I realized just how critically important it is for childfree adults to make sure we put energy into building a strong support network for ourselves. This can be accomplished in a variety of ways, including building closer relationships with neighbors and friends or getting involved in social groups or churches. We can also make sure that we are planning for our future by setting aside money to provide for our own care whenever we may need it.

If childfree adults are aware of this vulnerability and, as a result, build up strong support networks for themselves, they may actually be in a better position than couples with kids for a few reasons. For one, childfree couples and singles do not face the "empty nest" stage in life, and the time and energy available to devote to friendships is more consistent across our adult lives than it is for most parents. Second, the common myth persists that having children will provide us with support in old age. I recall a conversation Chris and I had a few months back when we were talking about what plans we might make for our older years. He said he expected that his daughter would be there for him. At first, I was struck with an immediate sense of fear, as I recognized that I had no one who would fill that need for me. But I then began to laugh aloud, as Chris's daughter lives in another state. She's quite independent, and she's likely to be even more so twenty years from now. I hear stories every day from parents who are disappointed that their adult children are not there for them, and sadly, no contingency planning has been done. Many

"Social connections and friendships are the most important thing of all in life."

childfree adults, like myself, have put significant energy into maintaining long-term friendships, and many have prepared financially for the day when they will need to hire the kind of support that some might imagine they will get from their children.

I have witnessed a number of elderly adults who are disappointed in the lack of support offered by their adult children and who have needed to seek out help from agencies or from younger friends they've met along the way. My ninety-one-year-old friend, Doug, is a great example of this. We recently hosted a dinner party, and Doug's daughter from California joined us. The conversation somehow turned to the importance of friendships, and Doug spoke openly about how much he appreciates having Chris and me in his life. He then made a point to express his disappointment in some family members who live nearby but seldom have time to spend with him. Another friend then began to share her sadness about her adult daughter taking a job out of the country, resulting in them rarely seeing one another. As the conversation continued, I thought about the words of wisdom offered recently by my father's cousin, Lyston, who is ninety-five years old and has one living daughter who is several hundred miles away from him. He shared, "Social connections and friendships are the most important thing of all in life." Cousin Lyston is especially close to my parents, his friends from church, and his neighbors. He is generous, and often invites people over for meals that he is fortunate enough to be able to still prepare in his own kitchen. In our society, we are becoming increasingly aware of both the importance of social supports and friendships in our lives and the impact of these relationships on our emotional and even physical well-being. Adult children are not always going to provide the emotional or tangible support that an elderly parent may need.

QUESTIONS TO CONSIDER

How strong is your support network? How might this be improved?

How do you anticipate having your needs met in your older years?

CHAPTER 6

HEALTH, FINANCES, AND FUTURE PLANNING

*"I just bought another $5,000 toy, a new telescope, and I'd
never have been able to do that if I'd had children."*

—Arno, age sixty

There's no doubt that being childfree has an impact on your physical health. On one hand, we have significantly more leisure time than most parents, but it's also true that our health may suffer because we don't have the pressure to be a positive influence on kids. Being childfree also impacts our financial health, including retirement planning. Childfree adults face unique challenges, such as finding ways to give to others and making decisions about our estates.

Physical Health and Well-being

Most childfree adults have the potential to exercise more, to get more sleep, and to plan meals more carefully, simply because of the significant time it takes to raise children. We ought to be capable of achieving better health than our peers with kids, if health is prioritized. When I compare my own life with the lives of my peers who work full time but are also mothers, the discrepancy in our exercise habits is significant. On a typical weekend, Chris and I go for a long run one day and then get out of town on the other to go biking or skiing. I don't think this would be feasible if I had kids, because I'd be thinking about all the things that had to be done over the weekend, including laundry, shopping, school projects, and children's activities. I'd have to put my children's needs above my own desires to have fun. I also think that if I had to handle the calendars of a child or two or three, on top of my own, I'd be overwhelmed. With kids, the skiing might not even be possible because of the expenses of taking the whole family to ski areas, clothing everyone, and buying snacks for the day. Once we arrived at the mountain, I might have to spend the day watching over my children rather than enjoying my own skiing. If the kids didn't come along, we'd have to find child care for the day—another expense—and I

"I actually think that I might lead an even healthier life style if I thought I was setting an example for my children."

would feel guilty about leaving them home rather than bringing them to a family activity. After skiing for the day in Canada, Chris and I like to stop in Vancouver for dinner before heading back home. The kids would be tired and we'd feel pressure to get them home to bed. By the end of the long day, I'd be exhausted from watching over, teaching, and listening to children as opposed to being able to enjoy myself. My physical and mental health would be put aside for the sake of the kids.

The childfree adults I interviewed had a variety of things to say about the topic of health and how they believe not having children has impacted them positively, negatively, or not at all. Laurie the engineer shared, "My husband Craig and I are both healthy people, and we have time to participate in sports we enjoy. Rather than watching or coaching kids in sports and various activities, we're out doing things for ourselves. I think it helps keep us young. We've developed a daily schedule that works for us without outside influence of kids and their activities, and this makes life simple. It's probably no major impact on health, but I believe our lives are less stressful than those of folks with kids." Another couple, Mark and Sarah, told me, "We have a lifelong habit of daily exercise, and our goal is to be reasonably fit and healthy. Among the people we know, however, being a parent doesn't seem to affect the ability to lead a healthy life." Mark smiled, adding, "I actually think that I might lead an even healthier life style if I thought I was setting an example for my children."

Jackie the paralegal spoke to the idea of setting a positive example from the perspective of a childfree adult. "I don't feel compelled to be a positive role model the way I might if I had a child of my own," she explained. "As a result, I eat whatever I want. I can come home from work and have three glasses of wine or ice cream for dinner if I want to without worrying that I'm being a bad influence on anyone."

Suzanne also agreed that she is no healthier than her friends who have children. She noted, "I believe that healthy choices are more related to self-discipline and time management than to whether or not a person has kids. I find that I often don't schedule time in my day for things that I feel I *should* do, such as exercising or meditating."

Denise, the divorcée in her early sixties, talked about how living alone has made it difficult to maintain the best health habits. She shared, "I feel better in every way, both physically and emotionally, when I exercise regularly. I could do a better job of prioritizing getting enough sleep and cooking healthier meals for myself, but living alone and having my second job interferes with having the time to cook balanced meals. I'm not sure that being childfree has an impact on my health, and I certainly don't think I'm healthier than my friends who have kids. All those women have very supportive husbands, and this makes taking care of exercise and diet easier."

Time and personal values seem to be the common elements here. If a couple with kids is financially able to have one partner at home full time, this may result in better health due to time for workouts while the kids are in school and time for planning and preparing healthy meals. Couples who both work full time, however, likely find it tough to make room in their schedules for a daily workout, and they may be more prone to eating meals out or picking up fast food for dinner. Childfree adults, due to fewer demands on their time, have more opportunities to maintain a balanced life.

Tracy, the self-employed web designer, talked to me about the concept of balance. "I make healthier choices because I have time. I definitely live a more balanced

"I believe I'm healthier than my friends who have kids."

life than my friends with children, who work full time and also have the kids to take care of. I exercise in the evenings, go out shopping, and then come home to make dinner for myself. It's easier for me to live a healthy life simply because I have more time."

Nicole the FBI agent shared, "I consider myself healthy. I exercise at least four times a week and sleep six to eight hours a night. If anything adversely affects my eating habits, it's my work schedule getting in the way. I firmly believe I have less stress in my life and am more rested than the majority of my friends with children." Elizabeth the marketing consultant told me that her health comes first, explaining, "I take care of myself. I have a good balance of physical activities and good eating habits. When my body desires sleep, I don't hesitate to sleep. For instance, on the weekends I often take a nap during the day or go to bed early without any thought or hesitation. I don't think any of my friends with kids have this luxury. I go to the gym and train with a trainer twice a week. I also do Pilates once a week and regularly see a chiropractor and acupuncturist in order to maintain good health. It's also important for me to make healthy food choices."

Diane, the accountant who tends to work more than full time, shared her challenges to stay healthy, saying, "I've had ongoing health issues for most of my adult life. I exercise regularly but don't eat very well. I also have a high-stress job. All that being said, I do believe I'm healthier than my friends who have kids. I've also noticed that coworkers with kids miss the most time from work either because of their own illness or the illnesses of their children."

Retired respiratory therapist Arno told me, "I haven't made the healthiest choices in my life, and this may have resulted in me now having a terminal disease. If I had been a dad, I wouldn't have smoked pot, because this wouldn't have been right. I don't exercise, sleep well, live a balanced life, or make healthy eating choices. I might have been healthier if I'd had a child."

Research on health issues suggests that certain lifestyle factors may result in childfree adults being healthier than parents. A study done by the University of Iowa College of Medicine and the University of Michigan found that adults who lived with children ate almost five more grams of fat and nearly two more grams of saturated fat a day than childfree adults, and they were more likely to eat foods such as cheese, ice cream, beef, pizza, and salty snacks.[17] This research seems to suggest that parents eat this unhealthy food because it's in the house for the children, but some parents talk about making unhealthy choices due to high stress. A good example of this is Martha, who came in to see me last year for counseling because she was feeling depressed and overwhelmed. She had a small daughter and felt guilty that while she was trying to teach her daughter about making healthy eating choices, she was gorging on ice cream and chips after her daughter went to bed. She took no time to exercise and was getting only five hours of sleep a night because she had too much to do in the evenings. Martha and I worked together on setting goals, but each week when she came in for her session, she'd been unable to follow through on the ideas we'd discussed. She said she simply didn't have time.

Childfree adults may also have better health than parents because they get more sleep. In a 2009 study in the Archives of

Internal Medicine, Sheldon Cohen, a professor of psychology at Carnegie Mellon University, looked at the importance of sleep in staying well. He found that people who sleep fewer than seven hours a night appear to be almost three times as likely to catch a cold as those who sleep more than eight hours, and that quality of sleep might count even more than quantity. People who spend as few as twenty-five minutes a night tossing and turning face more than five times the risk of catching a cold.[18] Children are notorious for interrupting the sleep of their parents, so it makes sense that not having kids would result in fewer colds.

This brings to mind Andrea, another ex-patient of mine. She was sent to see me by her employer due to chronic absenteeism and tardiness. She was constantly getting sick and feeling exhausted from not getting enough sleep. Andrea was a single mom and she had a truly hectic schedule that involved getting up at 5:30 each morning, taking her son to day care, and working from 7:15 until 3:30. She then picked up her son, drove him to his appointments or activities, and usually arrived home by 6 pm. Andrea then had to make dinner, help her son with homework, get him to bed by 8:00, and do the dishes and other daily chores. She tried to get to bed by ten with the goal of relaxing for an hour and being asleep by eleven. She'd start the whole routine again at 5:30 the next morning, on less than seven hours of sleep. Each week when Andrea met with me, we examined ways for her to cut corners so that she could get the extra sleep that she needed, but it simply was not possible. I remember laughing with Andrea about her impossible situation, and then telling her, "I'd last with that schedule for about two days, and then I'd have no other choice but to run away from home." One week Andrea came in and told me that she'd been fired from her job because she'd missed five days of work in two months due to illness. Oddly enough, though, she shared that she was actually happy about being fired, and that she'd spent the past few days at home alone resting and getting caught up on organizing her life.

Childfree adults also have the luxury of dealing with illness in radically different ways than parents do. A couple of months ago, I came down with my first cold in several years. I was able to get through the workday, but for several nights in a row I came home and lounged around all evening doing absolutely nothing and then went to bed at 8:30. I suppose I could have mustered up the energy to be productive those evenings, despite being sick, but it was nice to just relax. I also think that I recovered more quickly because I was able to get plenty of rest.

A topic that is gaining more interest all the time is the impact of stress and worry on health. I often think about this when I hear parents share their worries about their children. I recently heard that an old friend's young daughter has been diagnosed with a brain tumor. I can only imagine how much anguish my friend is feeling. Most parents encounter significant stresses with their children at some point, and this is bound to take a toll on their health. As the "mom" of a small, indoor dog, I can relate on some level. I recognize how much control I have over her safety, because Bella is inside all the time unless she's safely on a leash with me. Children, on the other hand, are out in the dangerous world and bad things can happen to them. Another friend, Linda, has a son who's now in the fourth grade. He's had some behavioral issues in the classroom and has even had to be moved to a new school as a result. I know from my talks with Linda that this has been a considerable source of worry for her. It begs the question of what the actual impact of having children is on your health, simply due to the stress involved in child rearing.

QUESTIONS TO CONSIDER

Do you make healthier or less healthy choices as a result of not having kids?

Do you think your health is better than that of friends and

colleagues who have kids because you have less stress and more opportunity to get adequate rest?

Financial Matters

It's no secret that children cost a lot of money, but many people do not take this into consideration when they contemplate having children. I was reminded of the huge expense of raising kids recently, when my old friend Joel came to my house for tea. He's in his early forties and has a new marriage and a two-year-old son, as well as two older boys from his first marriage. When I asked him how things were going, he talked about the joy of having three boys and how much fun he has with each of them, but he also talked about feeling financially strained, paying over $1,500 a month in child support for the two boys from his first marriage. As a childfree woman, it's mind-boggling to think about shelling out that kind of monthly expense when I'm supporting no one but myself and my little dog, whose organic food costs me $15 a month.

After Joel left that day, it dawned on me that he will still be supporting his son as he approaches sixty. According to the U.S. Department of Agriculture, families that make $70,000 a year or more will spend $260,520 to raise a child from birth through age 17,[19] and this doesn't include college tuition, which can add up to $150,000 more for a four-year education. This also doesn't consider lost income that occurs when one parent decides to stop working, to take off several years to raise their children, or to take a lesser-paying job with more predictable hours. I've seldom heard this taken into consideration when a couple is contemplating having their first child or adding another to their existing family. In my social circles and among my patients, the decision to have a child is more often attached to emotional reasons. I've heard people make comments such as, "We didn't want her to grow up as an only child," or "I really wanted to have another baby because I love the whole pregnancy experience and the first few years of being a mom with an infant."

Laurie the engineer shared, "Craig and I make good money and enjoy a comfortable lifestyle. There's not much in life that we want but are denied due to lack of funds. We have a good, well-funded retirement plan. Everything we own we actually own outright, including our home. I don't think we could have ever gotten this far financially this early in life if we'd had kids. I think a lot of couples are subject to a fair amount of stress due to difficult financial decisions. We never have to decide between automobile insurance or braces for the kid's teeth; between tickets to a Nickelback concert or swimming lessons; between a new motorcycle and paying for college. Knowing that there are no offspring who will take care of us when we're old and broken, we have to save now so that we are financially positioned to pay strangers to do that for us when the time comes. We are both totally comfortable with that."

Families that make $70,000 a year or more will spend $260,520 to raise a child from birth through age 17, and this doesn't include college tuition, which can add up to $150,000 more for a four-year education.

Elizabeth, the marketing consultant who lives with her partner, Maria, also works hard and enjoys the fruits of her labor. She told me, "Our money worries are different from those of my friends with children. I don't have to worry about college, schools, or even creating a budget. I think we probably spend the same amount of money, but we spend it very differently. For instance, I spend money on expensive dinners, an expensive gym membership, good wines, art, weekend trips at luxury hotels, and doggie day care, whereas my friends with children won't spend money on these things."

Diane also talked about financial freedom, sharing, "I'm an accountant and Patrick is a truck driver, and we're extremely fortunate when it comes to money matters. We have very little debt and earn good incomes. We certainly struggled some during the early years together, but I'd say over the past five years we have been able to live very comfortably. Obviously, being childfree, we don't have many of the expenses people with children have, such as child care and college, so we have more money for fun stuff."

Some childfree adults shared that they actually considered cost when contemplating whether or not to have children. Suzanne told me, "Not having enough money was a huge factor for me when deciding to not have kids. Also, John and I have always appreciated a 'footloose and fancy free' type of lifestyle, or at least the concept of it, and children need stability. We don't have a financial plan for retirement, and our finances have always been somewhat of a mess, simply because we've never had enough money because of moving around and sometimes working part-time. I've imagined that if I were to win the lottery and had millions of dollars, I might want to have a child. The funny thing, though, is that I can also think of lots of other things I would want to do if I had the lottery money, which would leave no time for raising a child. I haven't had to make the employment sacrifices that I'd have had to make as a parent. I feel like I have choices. If I had a child, I'd want to focus on his or her happiness, and quitting a job that I hated wouldn't likely be an option because I'd need the money to support the child."

For some single childfree women, money worries are a reality even without kids. Denise shared, "As an office manager, I haven't made a huge income, but I don't think my money worries are as acute as those for people with children to support because the cost of raising a child is incredible! I have only myself to think about. As a single woman, I earn quite a bit less than my friends who are married and have kids, simply because both husband and wife are working while I'm on my own. Because of their dual-income status, they are doing much better financially than me, even though they have children to support. I've never owned my own home, and at this point, with the drop in the market last year, I'm planning on working as long as I can. In observing the lives of my friends, I see how the financial obligation to children goes on and on. One of my friends has a handicapped child, and so not only does she have herself to consider, but also the long-term support of her son, even after she has died."

Nicole, also single and childfree, enjoys a lucrative salary and tells a different story. She smiled smugly as she shared, "My money worries are all self-centered. I don't have to worry about putting money away for college or unexpected health concerns for kids or school finances. I worry about which sports car I want to buy and if I'm going to treat myself to an extra week of vacation. I put away up to $1,000 a month towards retirement, and I also have a pension with my job. Financially, I feel secure. I only have to worry about myself.

> **"Being childfree has enabled me to put more energy into my career without having the added pressure of child rearing. I've always been able to work late or weekends without too much consideration for others."**

Being childfree has given me a lot of flexibility to buy things that I otherwise wouldn't be able to justify spending money on, such as a more expensive home, a new car, and electronics."

Not having kids means that childfree men and women are able to devote more time and energy to a career. For me, it meant having the opportunity to work long and irregular hours when I was first building my private practice or when I wanted to earn extra money. I see that my colleagues with kids tend to stick to a more traditional 9-to-5 schedule, while I've at times seen patients until eight on weekdays and on Saturday mornings. Now, after almost twenty years in private practice with no one to support other than myself and a head start on saving for retirement, I'm learning to cut way back so that I can enjoy being at home with my dog and involved with other kinds of work and play pursuits. Childfree adults are also more likely to view work opportunities differently than parents, who might feel burdened by these prospects. Jill told me, "I hear some people complain about having to travel for work. For me it's the opposite. If I ever have the chance to travel for my job, I enjoy it very much, while parents tend to talk about it with dread." This has also been the case for Nicole who shared, "Being childfree has afforded me opportunities in my job such as last-minute travel overseas that someone with children may not be able to take advantage of. I'm also able to work additional shifts, make extra money, and not have to worry about the additional cost of child care." Diane has also experienced this. "Being childfree has enabled me to put more energy into my career without having the added pressure of child rearing. I've always been able to work late or weekends without too much consideration for others."

QUESTIONS TO CONSIDER

How has not having kids impacted you financially?

Have you had more freedom in your career because of being childfree?

Discrimination

Some childfree adults report that they have been treated differently on the job because they don't have kids. Nicole told me, "I have been discriminated against because I'm childfree. I am frequently scheduled to work holidays, and one supervisor actually had the nerve to say this was because I don't have a family. I was paid 50¢ less an hour than a woman who was hired the same day and for the same job, and when I found out about it and asked to be compensated, I was told that the decision was made because she was a single mom. I also find there is a lot of leeway given to parents at work when their child is sick or has a school function or when there is no day care available. My supervisors don't care if my dog is throwing up; I'm still expected to report to work." Laurie expressed frustration with workplace benefits. She shared, "For many years Craig and I paid the same health insurance rate as a married couple with unlimited numbers of children. That was financial discrimination. The policy has changed now so that there is a separate fee schedule for couples without children." Diane shared, "I don't think I've been discriminated against financially for not having children, but I do believe that workplace parents, mostly mothers, are given more flexibility in their work schedules than women without children. The childfree woman doesn't have an *excuse* to leave work other than for selfish reasons while the mother is seen as leaving for selfless reasons."

The childfree adults I interviewed also expressed their views on the current tax structure, in which parents are financially rewarded for having children. In addition to a deduction of several thousands of dollars per dependent, many also qualify for a child tax credit of up to $1,000 per child. In some states, low-income parents are eligible for cash, food stamps, and medical insurance, while low-income adults without kids get nothing. These systems feel unfair to many childfree adults, who use fewer public services yet pay higher taxes. Suzanne shared, "I think that people should be financially compensated for *not* having kids." Jackie, the paralegal, agreed and added, "If I were to get sick, there is nothing out there for me. If I were, on the other hand, to have a baby, I'd be well taken care of. I'd have full medical benefits provided for me and for my child, as well as food stamps and cash. This feels very unfair!" Jackie went on to tell me about her bout with cancer several years ago, and how afraid she was at the time that she wouldn't be able to continue working and would have no way to support herself financially.

Denise viewed the situation somewhat differently, noting, "Having a tax reduction is recognition that having children uses more financial resources than otherwise would be the case. I think this tax deduction is valid, but other kinds of compensation don't seem as legitimate to me."

Annie noted, "I'm okay with paying property taxes, and I'd like to see free accessible birth control for anyone. Tax breaks for having kids seems fair because it does cost a lot to raise a child." After she shared her opinion, her husband, Roger, jumped in, proclaiming, "It's complicated.

> "I'm not real pleased with the tax structure. We have chosen to not populate the earth and those who have get a tax break."

I think the tax break structure should vary rather than being the same for every family regardless of income. In response to Annie's comment that it costs a lot to raise a child, I'd say that the reality is that it costs a lot to do lots of things. Why should parents be rewarded when so many other folks aren't? I'd like to be given a tax break for some of the things I'm involved in that are contributing to society in a positive way."

Laurie had an even stronger opinion on the topic, noting, "I'm not real pleased with the tax structure. We have chosen to not populate the earth and those who *have* get a tax break. When the country was new, it may have been necessary to create bigger families, but at this point it's completely illogical to encourage or reward having more babies."

I tend to agree with the opinions of Roger and Laurie. Sure, it's expensive to raise a child, but shouldn't this be considered prior to pregnancy? I believe that people should take responsibility for financially supporting their chosen lifestyle, whether this is making charges on the credit card, adopting a pet, purchasing a home, or having a baby. It doesn't make sense that a parent would expect someone else to help pay for his or her child's day care expenses.

Have you been discriminated against at work because of not having kids?

Do you feel that our current tax and benefits structure is fair? Why or why not?

A Desire to Give

It's a given that kids are expensive, but at times I've felt sad about not having a young person to provide financial support for, especially a child who is working hard to save for college or who deserves a special reward for reaching a milestone in life. At times I even feel a sense of loss because I don't have someone who is financially dependent on me, and I've come to see this as yet another human yearning that's wired into us as a means of keeping the human race alive. Once I became aware of this need, I began to consider ways I might be able to meet it. Being childfree allows me to choose to give financial support to whomever I want, whether it's a young person, an older individual, or even an animal—I get to choose who I feel is deserving of or most in need of my money. A parent, on the other hand, is obligated to financially support his or her children. The outcome of my brainstorming was a plan of action. I have since sent one hundred dollars to my college-age niece with instructions to spend it on whatever she wants. She's doing great in college and I want her to know that her hard work deserves a reward. I also gave several hundred dollars to our favorite waiter on his last night at work before he headed off to Spain to work on an organic produce farm. Although he's just in his mid-twenties, he takes his job quite seriously, and he recently shared with me that he has been working three jobs to save up for his European travels. I gave Ezra the card that night and he took a moment to open it there at our table. When he saw the four 100 dollar bills I'd placed inside, his eyes became huge and filled with tears. In the card I wrote, "As a childfree adult, I've set up a scholarship fund for young people who are going places with their lives, and you, Ezra, are the current recipient." Seeing the gratitude and surprise on his face gave me so much pleasure, and I felt fortunate to be able to contribute to his life in a real way.

Some of the adults I met with told me that they too have the desire to give to others in a personal way. Tracy shared, "I wanted to give money to my nieces and nephews for college, but now they're out of college. I might set up a foundation. I've thought a lot about it and now I just need to decide what to do." Nicole shared, "I have set up a college fund for my nephew, but I haven't told his parents. That way, if he winds up being a jerk I'll just have an extra savings account in fifteen years." Jackie has taken an active role in her niece's life. This year she took her niece on a Mediterranean cruise, a luxury that she says would never have been possible had she chosen to have children of her own.

QUESTIONS TO CONSIDER

Have you felt a yearning to "parent" a child or a young person?

What steps have you taken to fulfill this need? What ideas do you have for doing so?

Future Planning

Childfree adults have unique issues to consider when planning for the future. We are often better off financially, because we have the opportunity to save for our retirement during the years when parents spend enormous sums on their kids. Many childfree adults I talked to focused on the financial freedoms not having children has offered them. Tracy said, "I feel very secure. I have my own home and a healthy retirement fund. I feel lucky compared to my married friends with children, because if I wanted to, I'd be able to retire earlier than my friends with children." Elizabeth shared, "For retirement, I contribute to my work 401(k) plan, invest in CDs, have an existing retirement account, and contribute to a savings account. I own three properties as investments for retirement. I have a will, assignment of power of attorney, a living will, and a health-care proxy." Elizabeth is well prepared, and given that we are the same age, I realized that I have some catching up to do in my own retirement planning.

"I see an endless sea of possibilities. I can travel anywhere and live anywhere."

On a sunny spring day, I met with my friend Margaret. We sipped iced tea as she updated me on her life. Margaret is a fifty-five-year-old nurse who has been married to Richard for thirty years. Richard worked for years in real estate, but he decided last year that he was ready to retire. He quit his job and is now sailing to Chile where he and Margaret plan to settle. Margaret still works, but she's looking forward to joining Richard in Chile sometime next year. Not having kids has given them significant financial freedom. Margaret talked about how this has also resulted in a practical freedom—the ability to move to a foreign country, away from the town where she and Richard have lived for thirty years. She shared, "If we'd had a family, these children would now be grown and might even have kids of their own, tying us to them emotionally. My life would be focused around the grandchildren, and we'd want to be able to live near to them so we could be a part of their lives."

The reality of these family-type restraints was described by Jill, who noted, "I see an endless sea of possibilities. I can travel anywhere and live anywhere. Susan, my partner, already feels a bit stuck here because of her adult daughter who lives in the area and will likely stay around here. I'll also likely be able to retire earlier than Susan due to not having kids."

Although my retirement is not as organized as it could be, I have definitely experienced the financial benefits of not having kids. At forty-eight, I'm starting to contemplate making a career transition or cutting back on time in the office, and when I talk about his with my peers who have children, they simply can't relate. They're often still raising children or paying for college and haven't even begun to save up for their own retirement. If raising children is considered a career of sorts, then once the kids are out of the home, some parents might put renewed energy into building a career. If I view my psychology practice in the same way, after twenty years, it's time for a new focus.

This shifting of energy in mid-life is also happening with my friend, Marshall, who is fifty years old and childfree. Marshall earns a living as a musician, a web designer, and a day trader. Marshall and his wife of twenty-five years divorced two years ago, and afterward, he rented a basement suite in order to keep his expenses down while he decided what his next move would be. He then relocated to Florida, where he continued to do his various jobs. For Marshall, it's been important to have the freedom to travel, to focus on his work, and to grow spiritually, emotionally, and physically without being tied to children, a wife, or even a pet. I received email from Marshall a few months after he left for Florida, saying that things were going well. He was making new friends and enjoying the warmth and sunshine after years of Pacific Northwest rain. Many people would hear Marshall's story and pity him, thinking that he must feel lonely and disconnected due to not having the family ties of a partner, children, or even a pet. But if that's the case, he does an excellent job of denying it, as he appears to be thriving physically, emotionally, financially, and creatively.

Sometimes I fantasize about how I will spend my older years. In my fantasies, I'm often alone because of the reality that Chris is twelve years older than me and I'll likely outlive him. I used to imagine that I'd share a big, old house with some of my best friends. After Chris and I got together, I began to notice how involved he continues to be in the lives of his children, even though they are grown up. I also began to notice how common it is for grandparents to relocate in order to be near their grandchildren or to act as day care providers to those grandchildren. I felt some despair when I realized that, for my friends who have children, the parenting role would go on and on—I would never really have my friends back in the same way I did before they had kids. I realized that I'd likely not want to share a home with adults who have children and grandchildren and are quite focused on them, because this would take me right back to the place that I am now, with a huge part of our lives that we do not share in common. I've also noticed the emphasis on children and grandchildren when we've visited with Chris's mother, who lives in a retirement home. Whenever we go there for a meal and chat, the conversation among the residents is always focused on their children and grandchildren. I think about how awkward it would be for me to live in a retirement home filled with peers whose primary interest is their adult children and grandchildren. Who knows, maybe by the time I'm ready for a retirement home, some will cater to childfree adults.

In my conversations with other childfree adults, I found that they also have concerns about their future. Suzanne shared, "I think about the possibility of having to live without John, if he should die before me, and being alone. I hope that I'll have meaningful work, a social network, and the will to continue on with my life." Suzanne went on to talk about the poor job she and John have done of planning for the future financially. "Since we don't have kids, John and I haven't felt the urgency to plan for our financial future. We've tended to live for today, cashing out retirement funds as needed. I'm now reaching a point in my life, however, that I'm feeling some sense of need to invest for a secure future. Not having children means that we won't have the desire to retire for the sole purpose of spending extra time with children and grandchildren, as I've observed my own mother do. I can't imagine not wanting to always be involved in some kind of meaningful work, and I want to do a better job of prioritizing taking care of my health so I'll be able to continue to earn a living and to care for myself and my husband in our old age."

Nicole shared, "Planning for my retirement is just ensuring that I have a home and enough money in the bank to do what I want after I retire. If I had children, I would probably feel obligated to set aside a certain amount to pass on to them, and possibly their children. I haven't really done any estate planning, but I need to think about where I'd like any remaining money to go."

Jackie expressed her thoughts on the future, saying, "I don't think people should depend on children for their future needs, but I know it's very comforting for my mother to know that she has several people on whom she can count to help out. There's no guarantee, however, that your children will be there. Then there's the money. Parents mostly take on the responsibility of putting their children through college and that's money they might otherwise put away for retirement. I have my niece to leave my special things to. In thinking about what will happen to my things after I die, although I have my niece, I still feel really sad."

Portland engineer Mark noted that he sometimes feels that the option to rely on an offspring during his older years would be a nice option. "I also know that parents who are relying on that may well be disappointed," he told me. "Sarah and I have a fairly meticulous retirement plan with respect to funding, but we haven't figured out what we're actually going to do during retirement. We're planning our retirement so that our tombstones will read 'All Used Up.' We don't have any concerns about a legacy or leaving any money to anyone or anything specific. We do, of course, have a will that names beneficiaries in the event that we haven't used it all up."

For Denise, planning for the future is more of a challenge. She told me, "I plan to work as long as I can. This will probably at some point be part-time, but I think that with the cost of living and my financial assets, I'll need to work. When I can't afford to live where I am now, I'll move, probably to a low-cost senior residence. When I run out of money, I suppose I'll be the state's problem. This is where I see children coming in, because if one has a good relationship with their kids and the children have done well financially, they will likely help out their parents both emotionally and financially. I won't have that option, so I need to accept whatever might come my way. I'm lucky that I have my sisters and I'll probably call on them to be helpful in some way."

Carrie shared her experience of watching her mother take care of her grandmother. "I realized just how much care older people need. Someone has to love you unconditionally to bathe you and change your diaper or to make sure you're not neglected in a facility. I worry about this a little bit. My stepchildren love me, but not to that level. I can't see them taking care of me, but they might make sure I'm in a safe place." Tracy talked about how, because she doesn't have kids, she will likely be the child who's expected to step in to care for her parents in their older years. "My two brothers are married and successful, but I think I'll be the caregiver. They might help out a bit financially, but they have the excuse of being busy with their children and grandchildren, while all I have is my dog."

Some adults I interviewed also shared their thoughts on the bequeathal of their personal belongings. Roger the financial analyst married to Annie, shared, "We both have a lot of nieces and nephews, and I hope we'll be close to some of them as we age and can leave our personal things to them. We both like to work and we'll have money to pay for our care. Also, not having kids means that our financial picture is different."

Arno shared, "I will leave my personal things to my nieces. They will get everything. They're my sister's girls and they live in Texas and are twenty-three and twenty-one. I talk to my sister almost daily and she keeps me informed about their lives. I have quite a few family heirlooms, including my grandfather's cane and work tools, and a very old coin. When I hold it in my hand, I feel all those people from my past."

Childfree adults need to consider a number of things in planning for the future, such as ensuring there will be enough money to last a lifetime, which will cover personal care as needed. They also need to leave clear instructions regarding inheritance of their estate, and they should have a living will in place.

QUESTIONS TO CONSIDER

What kind of retirement planning have you done?

What are your expectations for your estate upon your death?

CHAPTER 7
FUTURE DIRECTIONS

*"I'm satisfied with my decision to not have children. Back when
I was married, my husband asked me if I wanted to have a
baby and I told him no. At that point, years ago, I was comfortable with the decision, and I still am. I know that I've
missed out on something in this lifetime. However, I can't
truly know what I never knew, which makes this easier."*

—Denise, age sixty-one

Life is all about choices and taking control over the things we can.
Childfree adults deserve to live the richest life possible without
being critiqued, and it's likely that the option to be childfree will
become more embraced by society as more childfree adults speak
out about their lives without kids. No one can predict the future,
but there are numerous reasons to predict that not having kids will
continue to be a growing trend.

Acceptance of the Childfree Path

For a number of reasons, our society is ready for a change, and I
believe that with each passing year an increasing number of adults
will choose not to have kids. As this option is brought to the surface
and talked about openly, more and more adults will consider not
having children as a legitimate choice. A similar societal acceptance

has taken place among gays and lesbians. Looking back a few decades, many homosexuals hid their sexual preference and their relationships for fear of being shunned by mainstream society. As a few began to boldly step forward to say that they would no longer live in the closet, more and more joined the ranks. Similarly, as more and more childfree adults speak out, others will feel more comfortable expressing their views.

Just as it did for homosexuals, the terminology for a childfree status is beginning to shift, and this makes a huge difference in how we view ourselves and how we are perceived by society. When I began to talk to other adults without kids, I discovered that even the simple task of coming up with a neutral term for our status was a challenge. Some referred to themselves as *childless*, despite their satisfaction with not being a parent.

> "When I hear the word *childless*, what I feel most is curiosity because I don't view it as a loss. I'm fascinated with the term and why anyone would want to refer to herself in this way. Childfree—I like that!"

Jill shared her perception of the term *childless* saying, "When I hear the word, what I feel most is curiosity because I don't view it as a loss. I'm fascinated with the term and why anyone would want to refer to herself in this way. *Childfree*—I like that! I remember stumbling across it years ago when I was in graduate school and thinking how much it resonated with me."

It's a fact that some people, parents in particular, find the word *childfree* to be offensive, as if it implies that kids are a nuisance. However, at this time, there simply is no better term. Even though this descriptor may offend some people, I choose to use it because my other options feel negative and focused on loss. As we become more cohesive as a group, perhaps new terms and language will be defined that have no positive or negative connotations. In the meantime, many childfree adults will simply say, "I don't have kids."

The more we begin to talk openly about whether or not to have kids and how to finalize this decision, the better off we will be individually and as a society. When I met with Victoria, the nurse in her late fifties, she shared, "By the time I was thirty-seven, I'd had several abortions because I never really sat down to decide for sure that I didn't want to have kids. My husband then went ahead with the vasectomy he'd been considering for years. He seemed comfortable telling anyone about his righteous choice to avoid procreation. Maybe it's all defensive bluster, but he claims he's glad not to have kids. I was probably forty-two or so before I could respond to the question of whether I had kids or not by saying, 'Oh, I was the oldest of eight kids and did a lot of mothering when I was young.'"

> "I had a tubal ligation when I was thirty-three years old, and it took me ten years to find a doctor willing to perform the surgery on someone without kids."

During Victoria's childbearing years, it was far less common to be childfree, and her inability to face this decision head-on was a common problem. I, too, wish that I'd been able to really decide, rather than sit on the fence until I reached my mid-forties.

Victoria talked openly about her experiences working for Planned Parenthood and the philosophy of the organization that only children who are truly wanted should be brought into the world. She shared, "'Every child, a WANTED child,' is one of the slogans that rings most true to me. Perhaps that's because it liberates me, somehow, since I never did get to a place where I WANTED a child."

As choosing not to have kids becomes more of a mainstream option, the medical profession will likely be more willing to provide men and women with vasectomies and tubal ligations at earlier ages. Currently, it is common for a woman who has not had a child to be challenged by her physician and even refused the procedure. This was the case for Nicole. She told me, "I had a tubal ligation when I was thirty-three years old, and it took me ten years to find a doctor willing to perform the surgery on someone without kids." You may recall that Nicole knew from an early age that she did not want to have children, and she never once has faltered in this decision. Nicole went on to say, "This questioning of me, an adult who had never wavered in knowing what I wanted, was an insult. I don't see physicians questioning young pregnant women on whether or not they are really ready to become mothers and refusing to treat them if they are deemed to be too immature. In my mind, this refusal to treat is another indication that the choice not to have kids is still perceived as unnatural. I only hope we reach a point where not having kids will be considered a legitimate option and not questioned so that other women won't have to go through what I did just to get their tubes tied." Reflecting on Nicole's words, I realized that many people still hold the belief that a woman is missing out on an essential life experience if she chooses not to become a mother. Decades ago I heard a similar claim about pets—that allowing your cat or dog to be a parent was a vital life experience not to be missed. But we have moved to a different place, due to an increased awareness of the need to curb the overpopulation of animals.

Mark the engineer spoke to this idea of societal norms, stating, "I believe that people do not always have children responsibly, that perhaps they believe it's something they should do or need to do to fulfill some desire. Clearly there are plenty of people who have children who are not good parents. I think the only way society could have a more responsible approach with regards to family planning is through education, and I don't mean education in the classroom, but education that begins at home."

Increased social acceptance of the decision to be childfree opens the door to opportunity for anyone considering this lifestyle. The childfree can determine how they wish to live life and decide what to do with the couple of decades that won't be spent parenting. Some will need time to grieve the path not taken and to come to a place of peace and acceptance. Quite a bit of research has been done on the way perception affects mood, so it makes sense that when being childfree is perceived as a loss, negative emotions, like guilt or shame, often result. There are actual steps that can be taken to aid the shift from a negative perception to a positive or neutral one, including using the term childfree or saying "I don't have kids" rather than referring to yourself as childless. Instead of feeling like victims of circumstance, the childfree may find it helpful to use a narrative psychology technique to understand the path that has led them to their childfree status. The process used in my interviews, in which the participants told me how they reached their current place in life and described the positives of being childfree, mirrors the techniques used in narrative psychology. I could see how healing it was for many of the interviewees to have the opportunity to talk about their experiences. Most of them were eager to embrace rather than reject their status, and many wanted to feel respected for their position in the same way that parents are. I've been amazed by the complexities of the stories I've heard. Victoria emailed me and said that she had finished working on the answer to question number one, which asked how she had arrived at her decision not to have children. She sent me her story, an eight-page narrative rich with emotion and complexities. I met with Victoria a few weeks later, and she told me, "It feels like a coming out in some ways, because the book is going to be published and it will give me a chance for my story to be told. Writing this allowed me to shift a lot of perceptions of my own story into a more positive light and to see the 'becoming' that was happening to me over time and why I had made the decisions I made. I moved from thinking of myself as 'not ready' and 'not measuring up' to a position of simply choosing a life without children. Writing out my story and the decades that have intervened has allowed me to put it all in a positive light. Through the years, I've felt incredibly pressured to become a mother, and it took a lot of resistance on my part to remain on the path that I felt was definitely the way for me to go. It was not what the people in my life wanted for me, because they truly felt that I was lacking in something they felt was so important—being a mother."

Erica Jong once wrote, "Surviving meant being born over and over."[20] I interpret her words to mean that she has gone back and reviewed her life story in order to seek a greater understanding and acceptance of paths taken.

For most, the natural tendency is to use healthy defenses, such as rationalization, to feel good about where we are in life. I feel it's important to take it a step further, to find concrete ways to embrace our lives and to make them as rich and full as we can. I've done this by spending lots of time soul searching and making decisions about where to put my energy. A few years ago, I sat down and began to draft a long list of all the things I wanted to experience before I die. This list included travel plans of all kinds and topics to learn about such as how to grow orchids. A few items were tasks I wanted to master, such as the art of baking bread. Now I begin each New Year by spending some time alone thinking about what I want to focus on over the next twelve months. Some items on my lists have included writing a letter a week, studying Spanish, making an effort to see certain friends who live far away, growing an herb garden, taking time daily to play my piano, and inviting more friends over for dinner. I try to limit the list to four or five items per year so that the goals are attainable. Compiling this list each year helps me to stay focused and keeps me from spreading myself too thin.

On a similar note, I read recently about the concept of voluntary simplicity in the writings of Duane Elgin. He learned about simplicity from Richard Gregg, who writes that the purpose of life is to create a life of purpose.[21] He advises each of us to consider what our unique and true gift is that only we can bring to the world, and once we have realized our life purpose, to then use this gift and to allow it to determine how we structure our lives. Simplicity is about a life of purpose. I believe that one of my purposes in life is to inspire others to experience joy and to take risk and to do so by being a model of sorts. I freely share my goals and the reasons behind the decisions I make in a way that allows others to see the thought behind the action. I also embrace the notion of exploring the world and growing and learning throughout life.

According to Henry David Thoreau, "The price of anything is the amount of life that you have to pay for it."[22] My exploration into others' processes and perceptions about living childfree, and my own understanding of how I arrived at my childfree destination, has taught me that we cannot have or do it all. We have to make tough choices in our lives. Most of us cannot train for a marathon, work sixty hours a week building a career, fully embrace the task of parenting a child, and be a nurturing friend all at the same time. We have to choose the direction we want to take our lives. There are no right or wrong paths, simply different ones. Parents must give up some other paths they may have taken had they not had children. Those of us who are childfree will never have the life experience of being a parent. Even for those who very much wanted to have children, but by chance or biology could not, there is no reason to not find purpose and fantastic enjoyment in life. Our mission is to embrace our life decisions and then to create a rich and full existence for ourselves.

> Our mission is to embrace our life decisions and then to create a rich and full existence for ourselves.

QUESTIONS TO CONSIDER

Have you struggled emotionally as a result of your childfree status? If so, what steps might you take to feel better about this?

Make a date with yourself to sit down and draft your list of the things you want to do before you die. Make it as long as you'd like and write it for yourself, as if it were never to be shared with another person.

Ask yourself, what is your unique and true gift that only you can bring to the world. How might you structure your life in a way that allows you to most fully use this gift?

Go back to that list of things you want to do before you die. Which are in keeping with your gift? How much life will each of these cost you and are you willing to spend that much on it?

Awareness of the True Cost of Parenting

I propose that a second factor—the more widespread awareness about the true cost of being a parent—will result in an eventual increase in the number of adults who choose to be childfree. By cost, I'm referring not only to the actual dollar amount, but also to the emotional cost and the sacrifice of time. An increased awareness of the needs that are met by having a child might open up conversation about other ways to fulfill those needs. For example, many of the adults I spoke with told me about how they meet their desire to nurture through giving to friends, having pets, working, and volunteering. It's healthy to recognize that the need to nurture is natural, but there is more than one way to do it. Victoria discussed her belief that there is a biological drive to become a parent. She explained, "People fall into having children without even thinking it through. The conscious part of our being is small compared to the unconscious part. This yearning to procreate is a life force that keeps pushing on us all the time. I've found ways to keep myself protected from this, including helping to nurture a friend's baby rather than going out and having one of my own."

Likewise, many people believe that marriages are strengthened by the arrival of children, but in fact the opposite is the case. A July 2008 *Newsweek* article, written by Lorraine Ali, explores the impact of having children on marital satisfaction.[23] Ali's article cites a book by Daniel Gilbert, *Stumbling on Happiness* (Knopf, 2006), in which the author looks at several studies and concludes that marital satisfaction decreases dramatically after the birth of the first child and only increases after the last child has left home. According to Pew Research Center, between 1990 and 2007, the percentage of people who said that children were very important to a successful marriage dropped from 65 percent to 41 percent.[24]

> "People fall into having children without even thinking it through. The conscious part of our being is small compared to the unconscious part. This yearning to procreate is a life force that keeps pushing on us all the time."

There is also the idea that being a parent will lead to a rich and happy life. Once again, research shows that this is not the case. A 2005 study by Robin Simon at Florida State University reviewed data gathered from 13,000 Americans. Simon found that no group of parents—married, single, step, or even empty nest—reported significantly greater emotional well-being than people who had never had children.[25] Arthur C. Brooks, author of *Gross National Happiness: Why Happiness Matters for America—and How We Can Get More of It*, found that parents are about 7 percentage points less likely to report being happy than adults without children.[26] These findings are certainly counterintuitive to the idea that children are the key to happiness and a healthy life.

QUESTIONS TO CONSIDER

How have you met your need to nurture?

How would you compare your marital satisfaction to that of your friends who have children?

How would you compare your individual life satisfaction to that of your friends who are parents?

The Environmental Crisis

I predict that a third factor, the environmental crisis, will result in more people choosing to be childfree. Since the late 1700s, when Thomas Malthus predicted that population growth would outrun food supply by the mid-nineteenth century, futurists have been speculating on the impact of population growth over time. Many of the childfree adults I talked to mentioned Paul Ehrlich's book, *The Population Bomb* (Ballantine, 1968), which was popular in the 1970s. This book was the inspiration for many not to have children of their own or to limit their family size to one or two kids. Articles on water shortages and shrinking numbers of fish in the oceans appear every day in the news. I personally feel a huge sense of anxiety about the future of our world. I question what people will be eating and drinking fifty years from now.

Victoria told me, "I thought about Paul Erlich's *Population Bomb*, which I'd read back in college and even made a speech on for one of my classes. I understood that when there are too many to support, some have to be abandoned or all will die. Erlich suggested that when some are damaged beyond a certain point, it doesn't make sense to use resources trying to keep them alive. It's better to focus on the sparks that have a chance to glow. I understood that life involves hard choices."

There is growing recognition of the toll that children have on the environment, and from that the argument has sprung that parents should not be compensated for having children. I predict that childfree adults will begin to speak out on this, especially as we become more cohesive as a group and as our numbers grow. In time I anticipate that people will be compensated for *not* having kids.

Many of the adults I met with shared ideas on this concept. Jill noted, "I think that there should be tax incentives for delaying having children." Laurie told me, "Pumping out kids is not something you should be rewarded for financially. Being DINKs [Double Income No Kids], our burden on society is much lower than that of people with children. Likewise, we both are full-time workers contributing to society, paying taxes, and social security. It doesn't make sense to me that people with kids get a tax break that we're not eligible for." Nicole noted, "I think most children are planned for, as most people want to start a family of their own, but I think the timing of most pregnancies is accidental. There should be more sex education available and family planning, and birth control should be available free of charge. I also believe that there should be free sterilization available for anyone after having their second child. There should be no compensation for having children. In fact, after your second child, unless you are adopting or fostering, it should be the opposite. There should be no large tax breaks, no additional stimulus payments. People need to be more responsible and consider the impact they and their families have on our planet."

> "Pumping out kids is not something you should be rewarded for financially."

I've thought about the idea of proposing a "take a break from sex" week once a year. If this were to turn into a popular worldwide concept, imagine just how many babies would not be conceived as a result. I strongly believe that the ultimate answer to our environmental issues is a decrease in population, and in order to have a true impact, this must occur on a global level.

Within the next decade, Japan and some countries in Western Europe are expected to encounter negative population growth due to sub-replacement fertility rates. Some governments are trying to find ways to encourage folks to have larger families due to concerns about lack of financial support for those reaching retirement age. As a society, we must be innovative and focused on building a healthy future. We need to explore ways to financially support older generations that involve new ideas other than having more babies to enter the workforce and pay taxes. There must be another solution.

Have concerns about the future impacted your thoughts on whether or not to have children?

What thoughts do you have on how we might ensure that there are sufficient resources for generations to come?

What thoughts do you have on ways to provide for the future, other than through having children?

The Childfree Tipping Point

As increasing numbers of adults choose not to have kids, more young people who are contemplating their future options will see that a childfree life is a respected and viable choice. Malcolm Gladwell's book, *The Tipping Point: How Little Things Can Make a Big Difference*, describes the way trends develop over time, starting as simple ideas embraced by a few and growing into epidemic proportions. He proposes that ideas and behaviors spread just like viruses do. They are contagious; small causes can have large effects and change happens not gradually but at one dramatic moment. At this point, the United States is gripped with baby worship. Every day there are articles published about celebrities having babies, and there are reality TV shows aired that glamorize large families. At the same time, though, another message is coming forward. We are shown how irresponsible many of these parents are and how their choices result in the damage of their children and to society as a whole. A recent example is the infamous octomom in California, who had eight premature babies as a result of in-vitro fertilization. This is a woman who already had six children, some of whom are disabled. An uproar swept through the country about the cost of this family to the state of California. Another case that is making headlines is the reality television show, *Jon & Kate Plus Eight*, which features the daily lives of a couple and their eight children. Jon and Kate separated several months ago, and now the show is focusing on Kate as a single mother to her eight children. Kate has shared with the media that her kids are acting out because they're feeling distressed about the divorce. The media tends to minimize how having children impacts marriage and how children are affected by their parents separating, yet there are just as many news flashes reporting celebrity divorces as celebrity births. At some point, all of this news is bound to create a backlash of negative emotion, if for no other reason than the parents' clear lack of concern for the children in these homes.

I am certainly not proposing that everyone should be childfree, nor am I anti-divorce, but what I am suggesting is that we, as a culture, begin to take responsibility for our decisions and how they impact our children and society as a whole. Once a child is born, his parents' desires have to be put on the back burner. If an individual is not certain that he is willing or able to do this, he ought to strongly consider not becoming a parent. I recall just recently asking a young father what his plans were for financially supporting his child, whom he'd had with a casual girlfriend. He looked at me with a sense of puzzlement, and replied, "I haven't really thought about it." Because the mother of his child is unmarried, she is eligible for state assistance, and since the father is not working, he is not even required to pay child support.

Another idea Gladwell discusses in *The Tipping Point* is The Law of the Few, which states that there are exceptional people out there who are capable of starting epidemics.[27] He also describes The

Lesson of Stickiness, which proposes that there is a simple way to package information that, under the right circumstances, makes it irresistible. What must underlie successful epidemics, in the end, is a bedrock belief that change is possible and that people can radically transform their behavior or beliefs in the face of the right kind of impetus. I believe that, as more and more childfree adults speak out with pride about their choice, there will be greater numbers who join the group. Up to this point, most vocal childfree adults have been perceived as negative and child-hating. For example, the childfree social group No Kidding! tends to be perceived as anti-children. My hope is that we, as childfree adults, will begin to be viewed as a group that is not opposed to having kids and that our life choice will be celebrated. One of my personal goals is to increase the size of this group of normal, healthy, nurturing adults who are not anti-family or anti-child. I have been pleased to see that some celebrities are beginning to speak out with pride about their choice to not have kids. Like it or not, these are the folks who hold social power and have the opportunity to influence others. If we can find and reach those few special people who hold so much social power, and if they can package their message attractively, we may be able to shape the course of a childfree social epidemic. Tipping points are a reaffirmation of the potential for change and the power of intelligent action. According to Gladwell, "The world around you may seem like an immovable, implacable place, but it's not. With the slightest push, in just the right place, it can be tipped."[28]

QUESTIONS TO CONSIDER

Can you envision a world in which the childfree movement begins to take hold?

Who are some of the exceptional adults who might start a childfree epidemic?

Creating Peaceful Coexistence

My hope is that we will soon arrive at a point where not having kids is as acceptable an option as having kids, and that we'll arrive at this place without a huge rift forming between parents and the child-free. We are indeed moving into a new era, following generations that have moved into adulthood and then automatically into parenthood as if this were the only

> "I like my life; I really, really like my life. It's full with things that I've chosen."

path to take. As the stories told by the childfree adults in this book reveal, many of us who don't have kids are, in many ways, quite self-indulgent. We have our own time, good health (if we choose to prioritize this), and money. For us, choosing not to have children has involved a recognition that not all roads can be taken. Taking time to examine whether or not to have children is a fairly new concept. Young adults entering the childbearing stage of their lives deserve to have the opportunity to explore their options and to be given validation and respect for whichever path they choose to take. Society should encourage everyone to embrace and to take full responsibility for their choice, whatever it is. As one childfree adult, Carrie, concluded in my meeting with her, "I like my life; I really, really like my life. It's full with things that I've chosen."

QUESTIONS TO CONSIDER

What are your thoughts on the concept of the tipping point, and how might this apply to choosing to be childfree?

How might we move toward a culture that embraces choice and do so in a way that does not split parents and childfree adults?

NOTES

1. Leon Festinger, Henry W. Riecken, and Stanley Schachter, *When Prophecy Fails: A Social and Psychological Study of a Modern Group That Predicted the Destruction of the World* (New York: Harper Torchbooks, 1956).

2. National Center for Health Statistics, "Birth Data," http://www. www.cdc.gov/nchs/births.htm.

3. Stanley K. Henshaw, Guttmacher Institute, "Unintended Pregnancy in the United States," *Family Planning Perspectives*, vol. 30, no. 1, Jan/Feb (1998), http://www.guttmacher.org/pubs/journals/3002498.html.

4. Cara Swann, "The Childfree and Pets," *Suite101*, June 30, 2000, http://www.suite101.com/article.cfm/childfree_by_choice/42395.

5. Associated Press Polls 2009, "AP-Petside.com—Pets and their owners," June 23, 2009, http://surveys.ap.org.

6. Polly Vernon, "Why I Don't Want Children," *The Observer*, February 8, 2009, http://www.theguardian.co.uk/lifeandstyle/2009/feb/08/motherhood-children-babies.

7. Polly Vernon, "It takes guts to say: 'I don't want children,'" *The Observer*, June 14, 2009, http://guardian.co.uk/commentisfree/2009/jun/14/polly-vernon-childlessness-cameron-diaz-babies.

8. Cameron Diaz, interview by *Cosmopolitan UK*, July 2009.

9. Christine Brooks, "Being True to Myself: A Grounded Theory Explanation of the Process and Meaning of the Early Articulation of Intentional Childlessness," PhD diss., Institute of Transpersonal Psychology, 2007.

10. Rachel Cooke, "The Dummy Mummy Decade" *The Guardian*, February 8, 2009, http://www.theguardian.co.uk/lifeandstyle/2009/feb/08/motherhood-children-babies.

11. Kirsten Dirksen, "Cameron Diaz on Her Childfree Status and Why the Planet Needs More Non-breeders," *The Huffington Post*, June 25, 2009, http://www.huffingtonpost.com/kirsten-dirksen/cameron-diaz-on-her-child_b_220582.html.

12. Nancy Rome, "Childless: Some by Chance, Some by Choice: I Lost a Baby—and Found A Community of Women Who Won't Be Mothers," *The Washington Post*, November 28, 2006, http://www.washingtonpost.com/wp-dyn/content/article/2006/11/24/AR2006112400986.html.

13. Steve Thompson, "Sex After Children: What Changes?" *Lifestyle*, August 18, 2006.

14. Cara Swann, "World Childfree Day," *Suite101*, June 1, 2001, http://www.suite101.com/article.cfm/childfree_by_choice/70159.

15. Susan Lang, *Cornell University Science News*, May 9, 1997.

16. Stephanie Coontz, "Till Children Do Us Part," *New York Times,* February 2009.

17. University of Iowa Health Care News, "Adults Living with Children Eat More Fat," January 15, 2007, http://www.uihealthcare.com/news/news/2007/01/15eatfat.html.

18. Sheldon Cohen, "Sleep Habits and Susceptibility to the Common Cold," *Archives of Internal Medicine*, vol. 169, no. 1, January 12, 2009, http://archinte.ama-assn.org/cgi/content/abstract/169/1/62.

19. "Raising your quarter-million dollar baby," *MSN Money*, 2009, https://www.moneycentral.msn.com/content/collegeandfamily/raisekids/p37245.asp.

20. Erica Jong, *Fear of Flying* (Texas: Holt, Rinehart, and Winston, 1973).

21. Richard B. Gregg, *The Value of Voluntary Simplicity* (The Floating Press, 2009).

22. Henry David Thoreau, *Walden* (New York: E.P Dutton & Co., 1904).

23. Lorraine Ali, "Having Kids Makes You Happy," *Newsweek*, July 2008.

24. Paul Taylor, Cary Funk, and April Clark, "Generation Gap in Values, Behaviors: As Marriage and Parenthood Drift Apart, Public Is Concerned about Social Impact," Pew Research Center, July 2007.

25. Robin Simon and Ranae J. Evenson, "Clarifying the Relationship between Parenthood and Depression," *Journal of Health and Social Behavior*, 46: 341-358.

26. Arthur C. Brooks, *Gross National Happiness: Why Happiness Matters for America—and How We Can Get More Of It* (New York: Basic Books, 2008).

27. Malcolm Gladwell, *The Tipping Point: How Little Things Can Make a Big Difference* (New York: Little, Brown, and Company, 2000).

28. Ibid., 259.

CHILDFREE SOURCES

Web Sites

IDoNotWantKids.com: a dating site

NoKidding.net: a worldwide social-networking organization

Books

Cain, Madelyn. *The Childless Revolution: What It Means to Be Childless Today*. Cambridge, MA: Perseus, 2002.

Defago, Nicki. *Childfree and Loving It!* London: Vision, 2005.

Dell, Diana L. and Suzan Erem. *Do I Want to Be a Mom?: A Woman's Guide to the Decision of a Lifetime*. Chicago: Contemporary Books, 2004.

Jeffers, Susan. *I'm Okay, You're a Brat! Setting the Priorities Straight and Freeing You from the Guilt and Mad Myths of Parenthood*. Los Angeles, CA: Renaissance Books, 2000.

Leibovich, Lori. *Maybe Baby: 28 Writers Tell the Truth about Skepticism, Infertility, Baby Lust, Childlessness, Ambivalence, and How They Made the Biggest Decision of Their Lives*. New York: HarperCollins, 2006.

Scott, Laura S. *Two Is Enough: A Couple's Guide to Living Childless by Choice*. Berkeley, CA: Seal Press, 2009.

Shawne, Jennifer L. *Baby Not on Board: A Celebration of Life Without Kids*. San Francisco: Chronicle Books, 2005.

ABOUT THE AUTHOR

Ellen L. Walker was born and raised in Jackson, Mississippi, and has lived in Japan, Maine, and North Carolina, before she settled down in Washington State in 1991. She received her PhD in Clinical Psychology from Seattle Pacific University and has a psychology practice in Bellingham, Washington. Dr. Walker and her psychologist husband, Chris, enjoy an adventure-filled life with their two terriers, Bella and Scuppers.

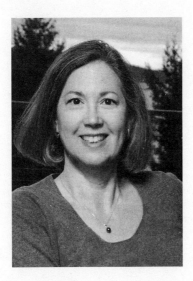